**Video Casebook:
Medicine**

Video Casebook: Medicine

The man who got lost in duty free

Andrew Levy PhD FRCP
University of Bristol, Department of Medicine Laboratories,
Bristol Royal Infirmary, Lower Maudlin Street,
Bristol BS2 8HW, UK

b
Blackwell
Science

© 1999 by
Blackwell Science Ltd
Editorial Offices:
Osney Mead, Oxford OX2 0EL
25 John Street, London WC1N 2BL
23 Ainslie Place, Edinburgh EH3 6AJ
350 Main Street, Malden
 MA 02148-5018, USA
54 University Street, Carlton
 Victoria 3053, Australia
10, rue Casimir Delavigne
 75006 Paris, France

Other Editorial Offices:
Blackwell Wissenschafts-Verlag GmbH
 Kurfürstendamm 57
 10707 Berlin, Germany

Blackwell Science KK
 MG Kodenmacho Building
 7–10 Kodenmacho Nihombashi
 Chuo-ku, Tokyo 104, Japan

The right of the Author to be
identified as the Author of this Work
has been asserted in accordance
with the Copyright, Designs and
Patents Act 1988.

All rights reserved. No part of
this publication may be reproduced,
stored in a retrieval system, or
transmitted, in any form or by any
means, electronic, mechanical,
photocopying, recording or otherwise,
except as permitted by the UK
Copyright, Designs and Patents Act
1988, without the prior permission
of the copyright owner.

First published 1999

Set by Excel Typesetters Co., Hong Kong
Printed and bound in Great Britain at
the Alden Press Ltd, Oxford
and Northampton

The Blackwell Science logo is a
trade mark of Blackwell Science Ltd,
registered at the United Kingdom
Trade Marks Registry

DISTRIBUTORS

Marston Book Services Ltd
PO Box 269
Abingdon, Oxon OX14 4YN
(*Orders*: Tel: 01235 465500
 Fax: 01235 465555)

USA
Blackwell Science, Inc.
Commerce Place
350 Main Street
Malden, MA 02148-5018
(*Orders*: Tel: 800 759 6102
  781 388 8250
 Fax: 781 388 8255)

Canada
Login Brothers Book Company
324 Saulteaux Crescent
Winnipeg, Manitoba R3J 3T2
(*Orders*: Tel: 204 837-2987)

Australia
Blackwell Science Pty Ltd
54 University Street
Carlton, Victoria 3053
(*Orders*: Tel: 3 9347 0300
 Fax: 3 9347 5001)

A catalogue record for this title
is available from the British Library

ISBN 0-632-05382-8

Library of Congress
Cataloging-in-publication Data
Levy, Andrew, Dr.
 The man who got lost in duty free
 Andrew Levy.
  p.   cm. — Video Casebook: Medicine
 ISBN 0-632-05382-8
 1. Internal medicine Case studies.
 I. Title. II. Series.
 [DNLM: 1. Diagnostic Techniques and
 Procedures Case Report.
 2. Diagnostic Techniques and Procedures
 Problems and Exercises. WB
 18.2 L668m 1999]
RC66.L48 1999
616.07′5—dc21
DNLM/DLC
for Library of Congress   99-24400
                                  CIP

For further information on
Blackwell Science, visit our website:
www.blackwell-science.com

Contents

Preface, vii

Acknowledgements, viii

Dedication, viii

Technical note, ix

Case Studies

1   The man who got lost in duty free, 1

2   A rash and a nasal voice, 4

3   A painful, hunched back and bed rest for a year, 7

4   Palpitations and unusual facies, 9

5   The man with a lump in the leg, 12

6   Ear pain, deafness and a trivial nose bleed, 15

7   The woman with thigh pain and double vision, 18

8   Lumps, bumps and palpitations, 21

9   Vomiting and collapse, 23

10   The man with the Rastafarian hat, 25

11   The hole in the gum, 28

12   Blackcurrant cordial, 31

13   Nausea and lethargy, 34

14   Intermittent abdominal pains, 37

15   A goitre and stiff hands, 40

16   The school nurse's daughter, 43

17   A television fault, 46

18   The tan that stayed, 49

19   A hungry, muscular diabetic, 52

20   Loss of libido, headaches and bad vision, 55

21   As smooth as a baby's bottom, 58

22   The perils of a 'lie in', 60

23   The man who couldn't mount a camel, 63

24 Spousal arousal, 65
25 A smaller cup of coffee, 68
26 Nasal discharge, 71
27 Facial flushing and abdominal cramps, 73
28 Recurrent haematemesis, 76
29 Weight loss and itching, 78
30 Jaundice and poor coordination, 81
31 The woman who giggled on the phone, 83
32 Slurred speech and choking, 85
33 An accident on the way to the airport, 87
34 Eye make up!, 90
35 The foot that flapped, 92
36 Dizziness and haematemesis, 94
37 Numbness, nystagmus and a drooping eyelid, 96
38 The man who couldn't let go, 99
39 Ear pain and facial weakness, 102
40 Muscle weakness and wasting, 105
41 Table tennis was fine, 108
42 The smell that wasn't there, 111
43 Breathlessness after a road traffic accident, 114
44 Progressive breathlessness, 116
45 A rash and stiff hands, 118
46 The man with a sore foot, 120
47 Recurrent gastrointestinal bleeding, 123
48 Episodic palpitations, 126
49 Refractory hypertension, 129
50 Cyanosis and breathlessness, 131

MCQ answers, 135

Index, 149

Instructions for use of CD, facing inside back cover

Preface

The ability to unravel the nature of diseases merely by listening to patients describing their symptoms is one of the most fundamental and satisfying skills in medicine. As meeting a patient face to face is more memorable than reading about a condition in isolation, this collection of 50 case histories is accompanied by the next best thing—a unique compilation of interviews and video footage of the patients on CD-ROM.

Impromptu interviews were conducted on a one-to-one basis during out-patient consultations or after ward rounds. In each case the handheld video footage of unrehearsed interviews conveys the real clinical situation and the patients' genuine interpretation of events leading up to their presentation.

The CD does not merely duplicate the material in the accompanying text. The video and sound files are complementary and unique additions.

AL

Acknowledgements

The author would like to thank his colleagues, particularly Dr Paul Taylor at Hanham Surgery, Dr Ken Heaton, Dr Ralph Barry, Dr Graham Standon and Dr Julian Kabala all at The Bristol Royal Infirmary and Dr Charlie Tomson at Southmead Hospital for access to their patients and their bemused hospitality.

The original camcorder and video editing platform were provided by Madeleine Curtis of Bayer PLC and Sandoz PLC. Dr Mike Stein from Blackwell Science had the insight to replace the camcorder after its untimely theft.

Dedication

To the 50 magnificent patients whose spontaneous goodwill and humour made this presentation possible; to my family, Ainslie, Rebecca, Hannah and Daniel, who put up with me, and to the staff of Blackwell Science who without exception were a pleasure to work with.

Technical note

The video and sound footage, still images and text were recorded, edited, compiled and produced in a book and CD-ROM format by the author. Video material was recorded using a Sony CCD-TR750 and subsequently a Sony CCD-TR810E Hi8 camera. Hi8 sound was recorded through a Sony ECM-55 microphone. Images were digitized using a Macintosh PowerPC 8100/100 equipped with a Radius VideoVision Studio™ board, JPEG compressed in real time and written onto a 4 Gb FWB Sledgehammer™ hard disc array.

Adobe Premiere 4.01™ was used for non-linear video and sound editing. Digital images were edited in Adobe Premiere and exported pict files edited with Adobe Photoshop 3.0™. Illustrations were generated using Adobe Photoshop 3.0™, Adobe Illustrator 6.0™ and MacDrawPro™ and then professionally redrawn for Blackwell Science Ltd. The CD-ROM presentation authoring programme was Macromedia Director 5.0™ on the Mac platform.

The introductory music *Longwave* was composed by Kaja May of Natural Productions and mastered in the Bristol University Music School studio by Jonathan Scott.

Case Studies

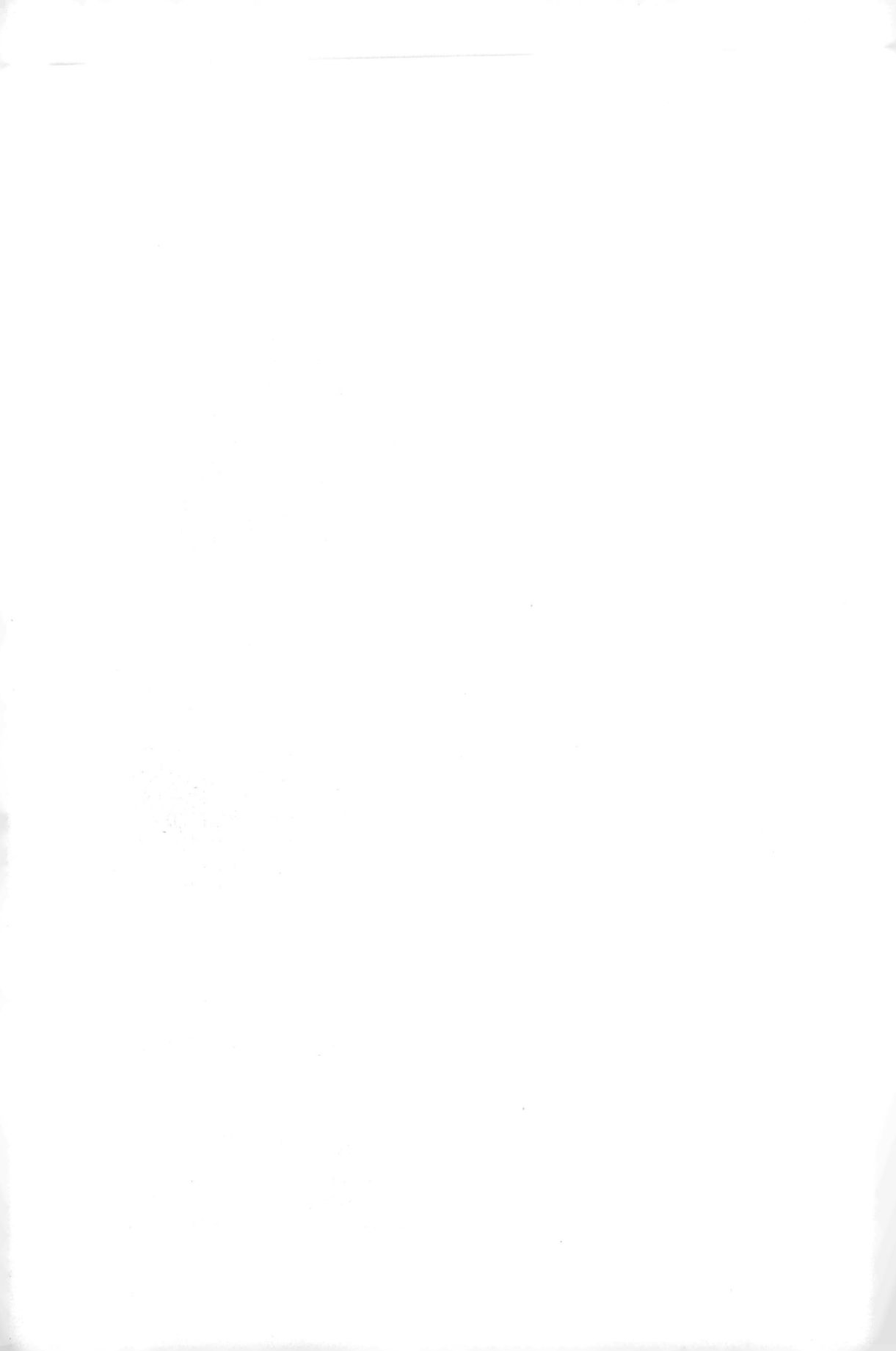

Case 1
The man who got lost in duty free

History

A 47-year-old gardener and former 'fan dancer' in various clubs in San Francisco was admitted to hospital with a short history of abnormal behaviour, loss of memory and weakness in both legs. He was a homosexual, single man who had lived a high risk lifestyle of intravenous drug abuse and unprotected sexual intercourse with multiple partners in sex palaces and bath-houses in a society that had a very high incidence of what was then called 'gay-related immune deficiency'. The diagnosis of human immunodeficiency virus (HIV) infection had been made over a decade earlier when blood tests for HIV became available and a skin lesion proved histologically to be Kaposi's sarcoma. From that time on, he had suffered from many of the typical complications of HIV infection with the exception of *Pneumocystis carinii* pneumonia. He had also had the sad misfortune to witness no fewer than four of his partners die from the disease. With a confirmed diagnosis of HIV infection and a somewhat reformed lifestyle, he decided to return to the UK from San Francisco and duly boarded the aeroplane home.

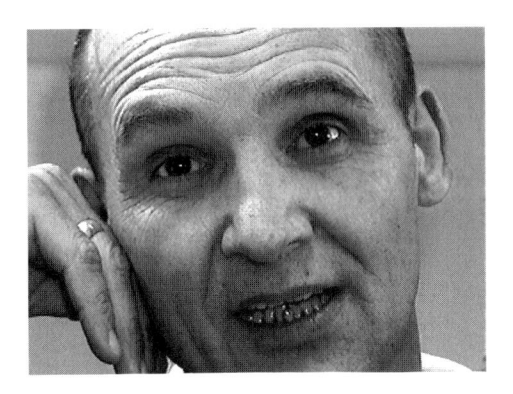

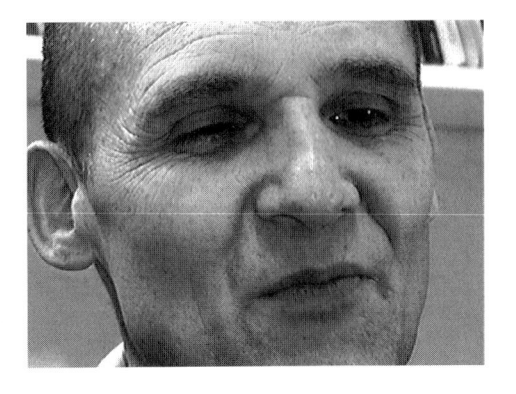

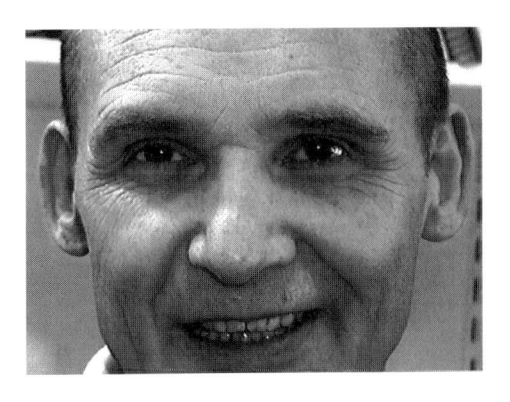

As he had assumed that his behaviour was beyond reproach, the patient was surprised and upset to be approached by the pilot before the aeroplane had even left the terminal and to be accused of being under the influence of alcohol. He was warned that if he did not behave he would be escorted from the aeroplane. In his defence, he explained that he had not ingested any alcohol at all, but that his HIV infection might have something to do with it. The aeroplane disembarked at Bahrain before the final leg of the journey, and the patient wandered off into the duty free with the other passengers. The first he knew of the imminent departure of the onward flight was that a stewardess had been dispatched to find him and wheel him back to the aircraft across the tarmac. On arrival in the UK, he was taken directly to hospital from the airport where other symptoms, such as paraesthesia of his thighs and a curious feeling that his knees were made of rubber, were elicited by medical staff.

Notes

The patient had acquired immunodeficiency syndrome (AIDS) dementia complex.

HIV is a ribonucleic acid (RNA) retrovirus, classified as a lentivirus, that is thought to have breached the simian–human species barrier near Kinshasa in the Belgian Congo in the late 1950s and from there led to the AIDS pandemic. On infection, the HIV viral genome is reverse transcribed by the enzyme reverse transcriptase (coded for in its own genome), and then integrated into the host cell genome.

Lentiviruses, which principally infect cells of the immune system, such as T lymphocytes and macrophages, cause many diseases in animals characterized by immunodeficiency and progressive wasting disorders, neurodegeneration and death. Unlike other retroviruses, the lentiviruses contain a series of complex regulatory genes that are thought to add to the pathogenicity of the virus.

The principal target of HIV is the CD4+ T-helper cell, because of the affinity of a glycoprotein component of the viral envelope (gp120) with the CD4 molecule. As T-helper cells coordinate a number of critical immune functions, almost all components of the immune system are eventually affected by the disease, and the clinical course reflects this.

Basic science

AIDS dementia complex

AIDS dementia complex affects about 10% of those with the disease, and is one of the most disturbing neurological complications of AIDS. It is characterized by difficulties in concentration and memory, apathy, motor dysfunction, poor judgement, incontinence, confusion and social withdrawal. When sensitive psychometric tests are used, a much larger percentage of patients with HIV are found to have mild neurocognitive disorder, resulting in impaired memory, motor function, attention, speed of cognition or language. Decreased serum vitamin B_{12} levels occur in up to 20% of patients with AIDS, and have been implicated anecdotally in the pathogenesis of the complex. The exact nature of central nervous system damage caused by HIV is unknown, however, but the neurological symptoms seem to correlate with the spread of the virus throughout the central nervous system. Interestingly, the new protease inhibitor combination drug therapies appear to be able to stall or even, as occurred in this case, reverse the condition.

Neurological problems associated with HIV

- Infections:
    Toxoplasmosis.
    Cytomegalovirus.
    Progressive multifocal leucoencephalopathy (infection with JC virus).
    Cryptococcal meningitis.
    Neurosyphilis.
    Tuberculous meningitis.
- Tumours:
    Primary lymphoma.
    Metastatic Kaposi's sarcoma.
- Direct HIV involvement:
    AIDS dementia.
    Aseptic meningitis.
    Vacuolar myelopathy.
- Other:
    Peripheral neuropathy.
    Myopathy.
    Convulsions.
    Cerebrovascular effects.

Pneumocystis carinii

Many patients with HIV infection die from other infections once the CD4+ T-lymphocyte count has fallen to below $0.2 \times 10^9 \, L^{-1}$ (normal range = $1-4 \times 10^9 \, L^{-1}$). The principal culprits are *Cryptosporidium parvum*, which normally remains localized in the gut, *Toxoplasma gondii*, which can penetrate the gut wall and cause systemic infection, and the usually non-invasive pathogens *Candida albicans* and *Pneumocystis carinii*.

Pneumocystis carinii was first identified in 1909 by Carlos Chagas, who also identified *Trypanosoma cruzi*. *Pneumocystis carinii* has long been known to be present in the lungs of most domestic and wild mammals. Nevertheless, the genotypes of *Pneumocystis* isolates from these hosts are so different that cross-infection between species is not thought to occur. Thus the sources of human *Pneumocystis carinii* infection have yet to be clearly established. Until the advent of the HIV epidemic, extrapulmonary pneumocystosis as a complication of *Pneumocystis carinii* pneumonia had been described only 16 times, always in severely immunocompromised patients.

Typical symptoms and signs of *Pneumocystis* pneumonia are mild fever, progressive dyspnoea and non-productive cough associated with hypoxaemia and hypocapnia. The chest X-ray typically shows bilateral interstitial shadowing. Definitive diagnosis is made by the identification of *Pneumocystis carinii* cysts or trophozoites in induced sputum or bronchoalveolar lavage fluid.

Trimethoprim-sulfamethoxazole remains the treatment of choice in patients with *Pneumocystis carinii* pneumonia. Different combinations of antifolate drugs are also used in cases of drug toxicity, and adjunctive corticosteroid therapy is indicated for patients who are significantly hypoxic ($P_aO_2 < 70 \, mmHg$). For the most up to date regimens, see 'http://hopkins-aids.edu/'.

MCQs

1. Cryptococcosis is the most common focal infection in the brain of AIDS patients.
2. Domestic cats and dogs are the primary hosts of intraintestinal *Toxoplasma gondii*.
3. AIDS dementia complex can be partially reversed.
4. HIV is a deoxyribonucleic acid (DNA) lentivirus.
5. HIV principally attacks the central nervous system.

Case 2
A rash and a nasal voice

History

A 49-year-old housewife was admitted with a 3-week history that started with the development of a dark, 'purplish' rash over her hands and face and the onset of progressive muscle weakness several weeks later. Three days after the start of the muscle weakness, she noticed that her voice was becoming increasingly faint and nasal in quality. Within 5 days, she was almost unable to make herself understood. Eventually, the weakness became so profound that she was unable to stand from sitting and was confined to bed. On further questioning, she explained that, 1 year previously, she had found a painless, non-tender lump in one breast. She had been too frightened to tell anyone and, untreated, the lump had gradually increased in size.

On examination, a mass, 3 cm in diameter, tethered to the skin and to underlying fascial layers, was found in her left breast, associated with left-sided axillary lymphadenopathy. By the time she was seen, the rash had resolved, but there was diffuse muscle weakness affecting all groups, including her bulbar muscles. According to the patient, at the time of interview, the abnormality of her voice was much less noticeable than it had been, but was still quite different from her normal phonation. A few vasculitic changes and dilated capillaries were present around her nail-folds.

Serum creatine kinase and lactate dehydrogenase levels were measured and were found to be elevated. A small amount of pectoral muscle taken at mastectomy and axillary node clearance confirmed the diagnosis. Electromyographic (EMG) studies were not carried out.

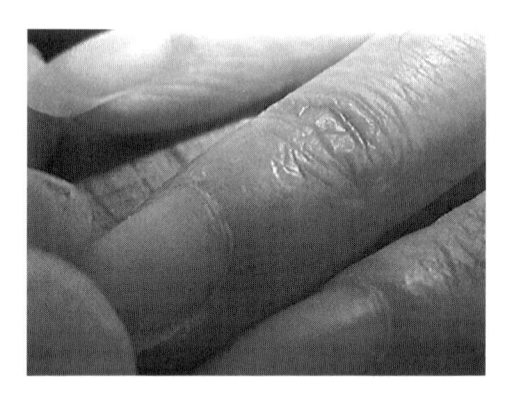

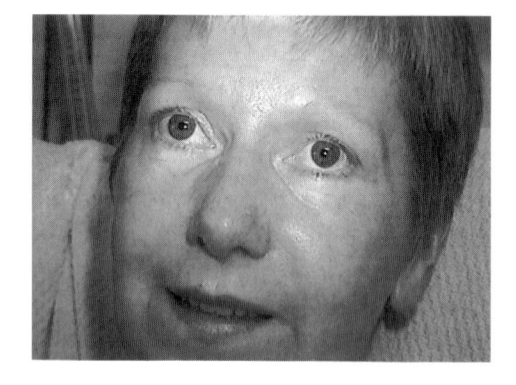

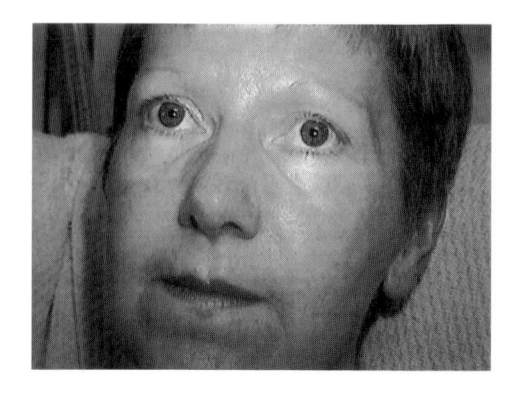

Notes

The patient had developed dermatomyositis as a complication of carcinoma of the breast.

Dermatomyositis is a condition of unknown aetiology, in which muscle is damaged by a non-suppurative, inflammatory process dominated by a lymphocytic infiltrate. The condition is characterized by a violaceous skin rash, which often takes the form of purplish periorbital macules (classically the colour of *Heliotropium* spp.) and purplish plaques extending over the knuckles and fingers. This change is accompanied by proximal myopathy and elevated serum creatine kinase or an abnormal electromyogram. Most cases occur in isolation, but about one-third are associated with connective tissue disorders and at least 10% with malignancy—most commonly of the lung, ovary, breast or gastrointestinal system. Dysphagia and respiratory impairment affect 25% and 5% of patients, respectively. The 5-year survival rate is 75% and, although at least partial recovery is usual, one-third of patients have residual muscle weakness. In the present case, the profound muscle weakness rapidly resolved after primary excision and chemotherapy for the breast tumour. The patient's nasal voice was caused by profound muscular weakness rather than damage to the cranial nerve nuclei within the medulla oblongata (the 'bulb' in 'bulbar palsy').

Basic science

Paraneoplastic syndromes

As antineoplastic therapy improves, patients with primary cancers are living longer, and the neurological and other sequelae related to the cancers from which they suffer, although uncommon, are increasing in incidence. In addition to cerebrovascular disorders, epidural spinal cord compression and direct involvement, such as brain and leptomeningeal metastases, patients with malignancy can develop remote or paraneoplastic phenomena such as peripheral neuropathies. The most common of these is a mixed sensorimotor polyneuropathy. In most cases, paraneoplastic polyneuropathy is thought to be caused by an autoimmune reaction against one or more antigens expressed by tumour cells and neurones. With the exception of the Eaton–Lambert syndrome, which mimics myasthenia gravis by downregulating voltage-gated calcium channels at the presynaptic nerve terminal, the mechanisms of paraneoplastic polyneuropathy for the most part remain conjectural. Antineoplastic agents, such as cisplatin, taxanes and the vinca alkaloids, are themselves potentially neurotoxic, and suramin can be responsible for a specific demyelinating polyradiculoneuropathy. In patients over 50 years of age, subacute cerebellar degeneration is paraneoplastic in origin in 50% of cases. Other paraneoplastic phenomena include acanthosis nigricans, thrombophlebitis migrans, necrolytic migratory erythema and erythema gyratum repens. Less specific dermatoses include exfoliative dermatitis, generalized pruritus and bullous disorders.

Speech

The symptoms that finally persuaded the patient to seek help were dysphagia and dysarthria related to the rapid development of bulbar palsy.

Aside from the purely intellectual and linguistic prerequisites, the anatomical, muscular and neuronal integrity of the respiratory, laryngeal and articulatory systems must be intact for normal speech to occur.

The diagnosis of speech disturbance caused by cerebrovascular accidents affecting large areas of the motor or sensory cortex is usually clear from associated motor and sensory signs.

Corticobulbar fibres carrying motor speech from the cortex to the IXth, Xth and XIIth cranial nerve nuclei in the medulla oblongata via the posterior limb of the internal capsule (just behind the genu) can be damaged by local insults, such as demyelination and microvascular disease. As innervation is bilateral, the sudden onset of impaired speech, chewing and swallowing, known as pseudobulbar palsy, does not occur until corticobulbar fibres from both hemispheres are damaged. Pseudobulbar palsy is associated with a small, spastic tongue in keeping with its upper motor neurone aetiology. Speech is said to be 'Donald Duck like'.

Bulbar palsy, lower motor neurone weakness of the IXth, Xth and XIIth cranial nerves, is a rare condition caused typically by motor neurone disease or acute idiopathic polyneuritis (Guillain–Barré syndrome). The tongue is flaccid and fasciculating, and the voice nasal owing to palatal weakness.

MCQs

1 Most cases of dermatomyositis are associated with underlying malignancy.
2 Dermatomyositis is associated with a typical skin rash.
3 In pseudobulbar palsy, the tongue is small and spastic.
4 A raised circulating creatine kinase level is characteristic of dermatomyositis.
5 Recovery from dermatomyositis is almost always complete.

Case 3
A painful, hunched back and bed rest for a year

History

A 65-year-old housewife and former factory worker was admitted with an episode of exercise-induced chest pain. She had a short history of angina pectoris diagnosed on the basis of episodic tight chest pain radiating to the left arm and face which came on after exercise and was relieved by sublingual glyceryl trinitrate (GTN) within 10 min. As the symptoms seemed to be worsening in severity, she was admitted for further investigations and for her antianginal medication to be optimized. On direct questioning, it became clear that her principal medical problem, far from ischaemic heart disease, was related to a gradual increase in breathlessness over the years and that chest infections, when they occurred, left her short of breath at rest. Her past history was dominated by orthopaedic procedures to her back following the development of severe backache and progressive kyphosis in her late teenage years. She had suffered with back pain for 6 or 7 years before the changes to the shape of her spine became apparent. After an operation to 'put it right', she was committed to bed rest for a year and then had a bone graft to bring about spinal fusion. The effects of the condition on her life subsequently were as profound as the effect on the shape of her back.

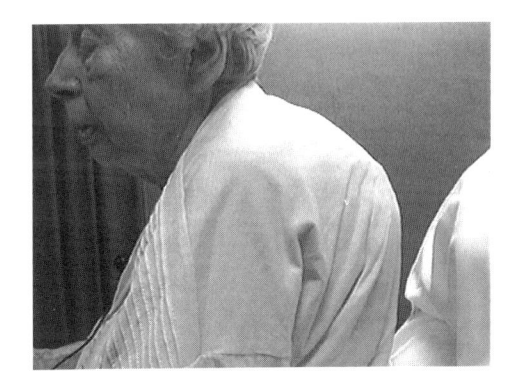

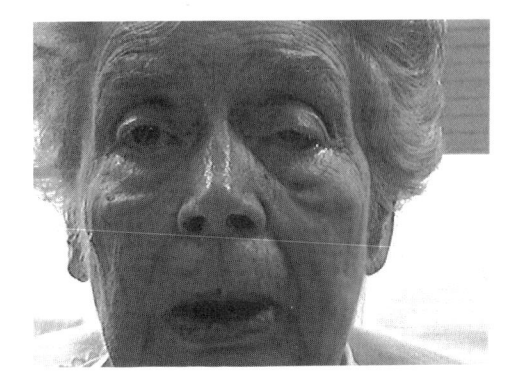

Notes

As a young girl the patient had suffered from spinal tuberculosis.

Pott's disease is tuberculosis of the spine. The sacroiliac joints and the mid-thoracic spine are typically involved, and the infection is thought to be carried in the bloodstream or through lymphatics running from the pleural space to the paravertebral lymph nodes. Reactive muscle spasm and truncal rigidity are accompanied by erosion of the vertebral bodies, leading to their collapse and the formation of a gibbus, a sharply angulated kyphosis. Antituberculous chemotherapy and orthopaedic or neurosurgical intervention may be required to stabilize the deformity, as they were in this case. Paravertebral abscesses are frequently associated with tuberculous spinal involvement.

Involvement of the bones or joints occurs in 1–3% of all cases of tuberculosis. In one-half of these, pulmonary tuberculosis is also present, and bone and joint involvement is the result of haematological spread or contiguous spread from, for example, an affected lymph node or from reactivation of previous disease. Typical symptoms are slowly progressive malaise and weight loss, fever, lethargy and localized pain in a bone or joint, such as the femur or ankle.

Basic science

Pleurisy, pericarditis and peritonitis

When the pleural space is seeded with *Mycobacterium tuberculosis*, pleurisy and a pleural exudate result, often with a fairly abrupt onset of pain. The presence of granulomas in a pleural biopsy is diagnostic. Pericarditis may occur as an extension of pleurisy or by seeding from a local lymph node. Peritonitis with ascites usually develops insidiously. Isolation of the organism from the exudate is often troublesome, and the diagnosis is difficult to establish. In the plastic form of mycobacterial peritonitis, the peritoneum is obliterated by fibrous tissue and adhesions.

Spinal cord compression

A locus of spinal osteomyelitis invisible on plain X-ray can lead to the formation of an abscess that enlarges rapidly to compress the spinal cord. The only symptoms may be a pyrexia of unknown origin and mild backache with local tenderness, leading to pain affecting a nerve root or complete cord transection syndrome. Even after surgical decompression and antibiotic treatment, local fibrous changes may continue to cause compressive symptoms.

Approximately one-half of all cases of spinal cord compression are secondary to vertebral disorders, such as acute intervertebral disc herniation or vertebral collapse. Typical causes of vertebral collapse are infections, such as tuberculous osteomyelitis, or neoplastic infiltration with myelomatosis or prostatic carcinoma secondaries. The remaining 50% are caused by intradural lesions, such as meningiomas or neurofibromas, or disorders of the spinal cord itself, for example gliomas or ependymomas. These causes of spastic paraparesis have to be distinguished from multiple sclerosis, parasagittal cranial meningioma (i.e. a meningioma of the falx, compressing the motor cortex on either side), transverse myelitis, anterior spinal artery thrombosis and motor neurone disease.

The Brown-Séquard syndrome, produced by hemisection of the spinal cord, consists of ipsilateral paralysis below the lesion (i.e. a monoplegia or hemiplegia depending on the level), ipsilateral loss of proprioception and vibration sense (as this is subserved by the posterior (dorsal) columns which remain ipsilateral below the brain stem) and contralateral loss of pain and temperature sensation (caused by section of the spinothalamic tracts) often one or two segments below the level of the lesion, as the spinothalamic fibres decussate one or two segments above their synapse with the sensory neurones in the dorsal horn.

MCQs

1. Hemisection of the spinal cord produces contralateral paralysis.
2. Hemisection of the spinal cord produces contralateral loss of vibration and proprioception.
3. Involvement of the mid-thoracic spine is typical of spinal tuberculosis.
4. One in five cases of pulmonary tuberculosis are complicated by bony involvement.
5. Around one-half of all cases of spinal cord compression are due to vertebral disorders.

Case 4
Palpitations and unusual facies

History

A 22-year-old student was admitted to hospital with a long history of cardiac problems, culminating in episodes of palpitations occurring with increasing frequency since a mitral valve replacement 3 years previously. For the 6 months before admission, the palpitations, characterized by runs of fast and very slow heart beats associated with faintness, had been particularly troublesome.

The heart problem was first identified at the time of admission to hospital for repair of a cleft palate at the age of 3 years. Surgery to close an almost complete ostium primum atrial septal defect left pre-existing clefts in the anterior leaflet of the mitral valve and superior leaflet of the tricuspid valve. Over the subsequent decade, these defects led to increasing mitral regurgitation and pulmonary hypertension. Symptomatically, the patient had become increasingly tired, with progressive exercise limitation, shortness of breath on exertion and orthopnoea. Insertion of the prosthetic mitral valve stabilized her symptoms of heart failure, but was followed by a tendency to episodes of atrial fibrillation and supraventricular tachycardia. The purpose of the current admission was to insert a pacemaker. The patient was noted to have rather unusual facial characteristics.

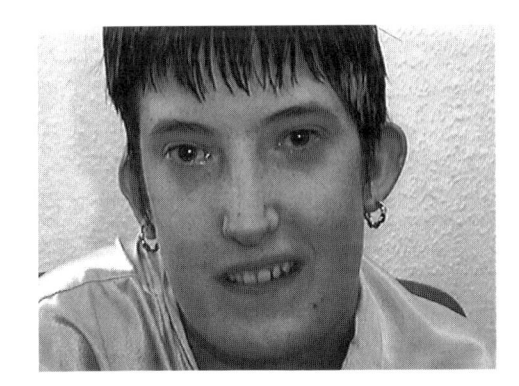

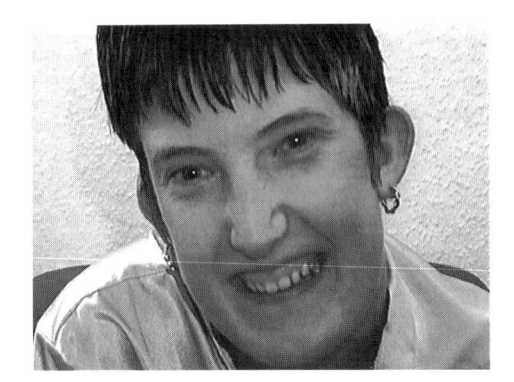

Notes

The patient's primary underlying problem was Shprintzen's syndrome. Shprintzen's syndrome, defined in 1981 by Goldberg and Shprintzen, is a relatively common syndrome, initially thought to consist of short segment Hirschsprung's disease, cleft palate and microcephaly.

Shprintzen's syndrome is now thought to be chromosomally closely related to Di George's syndrome, which was identified several years earlier, and, because of their common characteristics, the more descriptive term velocardiofacial syndrome is now used to encompass both. The common microdeletion of chromosome 22 (22q11) produces a wide variety of birth defects, including characteristic facies consisting of almond-shaped eyes, wide nose, small ears, a shortened philtrum and hypertelorism, and a tendency to palatal weakness and submucous clefting. Patients are predisposed to scoliosis and to multiple cardiac anomalies, including ventricular septal defects, right-sided aortic arch, tetralogy of

Fallot and aberrant left subclavian artery. Velocardiofacial syndrome should be considered in all children with cleft palate, in whom the syndrome is particularly common.

Basic science

Chromosomal disorders are mistakenly thought to be rare, perhaps because they are little discussed. The exact prevalence of velocardiofacial syndrome is poorly defined as the syndrome often goes unrecognized. Nevertheless, to put the epidemiology of chromosomal disorders into perspective, it is worth remembering that, for example, the incidence of Turner's syndrome is 500 times greater than that of Cushing's disease (pituitary-dependent Cushing's syndrome) and more than 150 times that of acromegaly.

The current patient's principal problems were related to structural and functional cardiovascular anomalies. Her admission to hospital was to address the problem of persistent palpitations.

Causes of sinus tachycardia

- Decreased activity (stretch) of baroreceptors.
- Inspiration.
- Hypoxia.
- Exercise.
- Sympathomimetics (adrenaline (epinephrine) and noradrenaline (norepinephrine)).
- Thyroid hormones.
- Fever.
- Pain.
- Excitement and anger.
- Anticholinergic drugs.

Causes of sinus bradycardia

- Increased baroreceptor activity.
- Expiration.
- Parasympathetic stimulation (e.g. 'vasovagal').
- Parasympathomimetics.
- Raised intracranial pressure.

Table 4.1 Other common chromosomal disorders

Syndrome	Karyotype	Incidence	Features
Klinefelter's	47,XXY	1:500	Male hypogonadism with small, firm testes, azoospermia (or oligospermia in the mosaic forms), gynaecomastia and eunuchoid habitus with increased stature and slightly decreased IQ
Down's	Trisomy 21	1:650	Round face with slanting eyes, epicanthic folds, small head, mental retardation, short stature, broad hands with a single palmar crease and short and inwardly curved little fingers. Congenital heart lesions are relatively common
XYY male	47,XYY	1:1000	Above average stature, mild mental retardation
Turner's	45,XO	1:2000	Short stature (rarely over 1.3 m untreated), amenorrhoea, absent breast development, renal and cardiac anomalies (50% bicuspid aortic valve, 10% coarctation) and osteoporosis. Audiological abnormalities are present in 90%, with a 30–70 dB reduction at 2 kHz (hearing of a 70 year old at the age of 40 years)
Edwards'	Trisomy 18	1:3000	Narrow, characteristic face with overlapping digits, multiple internal anomalies, severe mental and physical handicap and high mortality
Patau's	Trisomy 13	1:5000	Polydactyly, midline craniofacial defects and hypertelorism, cleft lip and palate, congenital heart disease, mental retardation and high mortality

- Sympathetic blockade (β_1-adrenoreceptor blockade).

MCQs

1 Resting heart rate is controlled principally by sympathetic tone.
2 The vasomotor centre, controlling the heart rate and blood pressure, is found in the brain stem.
3 Sinus bradycardia is induced by expiration.
4 The dorsal motor nucleus of the vagus receives afferents from stretch receptors in the aortic arch and carotid sinus.
5 Sinus tachycardia is caused by anticholinergic drugs.

Case 5
The man with a lump in the leg

History

A 76-year-old professional musician with non-insulin-dependent diabetes, who had smoked heavily for many years, presented to his general practitioner (GP) having noticed a painless, soft mass that appeared to be embedded in the muscle of his left thigh. No diagnosis was made, and the patient was reassured. The mass, which was several centimetres long, but barely raised above the surface of the skin, continued to grow and, with increasing concern, the patient went to see a physiotherapist friend who suggested that he seek a second opinion. By the time he was seen, almost 3 months had passed, and the mass, which remained painless, had increased to the size of a rugby ball. At surgery, the mass was removed and the patient believed that the problem had been cleared. Unfortunately, during surgery, the patient became hypotensive and suffered acute tubular necrosis which necessitated haemodialysis for a considerable time. He recovered over a period of several months and returned to his job. One year after his initial surgery, he noticed a small mass at one end of the original incision scar on his thigh, and was informed after biopsy that the problem had recurred. He was given 6 months to live unless the site was cleared by amputation. This procedure was duly carried out.

Notes

The patient had developed a high grade, soft tissue sarcoma of his thigh.

Most soft tissue sarcomas present as a painless mass without any associated symptoms, such as weight loss, fever or anaemia. Any soft tissue swelling beneath the deep fascia should be considered as a sarcoma until proven otherwise, and any soft tissue can be involved as the names chondrosarcoma, leiomyosarcoma, liposarcoma, haemangiosarcoma, myosarcoma, lymphangiosarcoma, fibrosarcoma, osteosarcoma and rhabdomyosarcoma suggest.

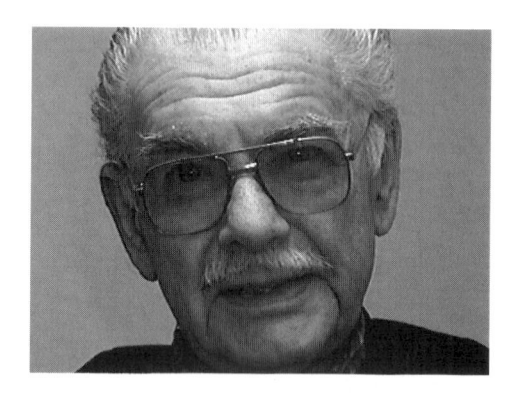

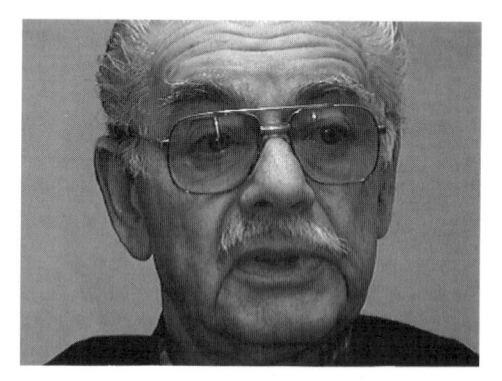

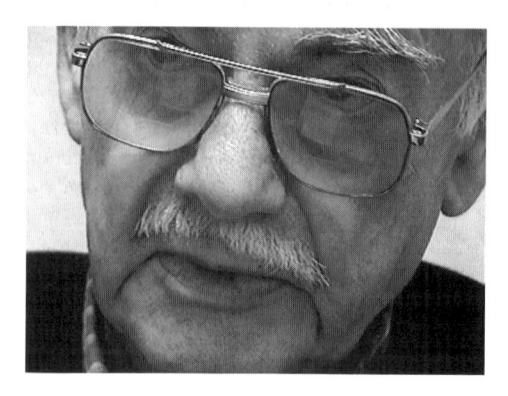

Soft tissue sarcoma accounts for ≈1% of all cancers and, even when Kaposi's sarcoma is excluded, the incidence has been increasing for many years. Aetiologic factors include external radiation, industrial mutagens, immunosuppressive and antimitotic drugs, anabolic steroids, human immunodeficiency virus and some herpes viruses. Inherited tumour syndromes, such as retinoblastoma, polyposis coli, neurofibromatosis and multiple endocrine neoplasia, also predispose to soft tissue sarcoma formation. The most important prognostic factors in soft tissue sarcoma are histological tumour grade and the extent of disease at the time of diagnosis. The most critical treatment is adequate primary surgical resection. Metastases develop in 10–25% of patients within 18 months of primary presentation. The overall 5-year survival rate is 75%, and 50% of patients can be expected to die from their condition.

Basic science

Inherited problems of connective tissue

Connective tissues are the extracellular elements that provide the structural support of the body and bind together its cells, organs and tissues. In addition to connective tissue structures, such as bone, skin, tendons, ligaments, cartilage and vascular elements, the connective tissues also consist of a matrix of proteoglycans and collagen fibrils in a plasma filtrate that contains about half of the total body albumin. Differences in the structural behaviour of connective tissues depend largely on differences in the size and orientation of the collagen fibrils they contain. Tendons contain thick, parallel, fibre bundles. In skin, the fibres are more random and, in bone, they form an orderly architecture around haversian canals, made rigid by the presence of hydroxyapatite.

Marfan's syndrome. Marfan's syndrome is an autosomal dominant disorder with a prevalence of 1:5000. New mutations account for 15–30% of cases, and the diagnosis is associated with a reduction in life expectancy, usually brought about by the development of aortic and mitral valve incompetence, proximal aortic aneurysms or dissection of the ascending aorta. The diagnosis is based around the identification of characteristic Marfan's involvement of three organ systems, including major manifestations in two.

The mutations responsible affect the fibrillin gene on chromosome 15. Fibrillin is an extracellular matrix protein that is a major component of the microfibrils found widely distributed in mesenchymal tissue. The most widely affected tissues are those containing the largest proportion of these structural elements, such as the great blood vessels, the skeleton and the suspensory ligaments of the lens of the eye. Typical features of the disease are dislocation of the lens of the eye, best seen with a slit lamp, the typical tall, thin body habitus and dilatation or dissection of the ascending aorta.

Lumbosacral dural ectasia is seen in 63% of those with Marfan's syndrome. Minor features are pectus excavatum, a high arched palate with crowded teeth, hypermobility of the joints, mitral valve prolapse, a tendency to spontaneous pneumothorax, striae and recurrent herniae.

The manifestations of Marfan's syndrome include the following:
- Skeletal:
  Disproportionately tall stature.
  Excessive arm span (eunuchoid habitus).
  Hyperextensibility of the thumb and fingers.
  Pectus carinatum.
  Pectus excavatum.
  Pes planus.
  Protrusio acetabulae.
  Scoliosis or spondylolisthesis.
- Ocular:
  Ectopia lentis (the lens is usually displaced upwards, leaving the iris unsupported and tremulous—iridodonesis).
- Cardiovascular:
  Dilatation of the ascending aorta.
  Dissection of the ascending aorta.

- Central nervous system:
    Lumbosacral dural ectasia.

Several other conditions have some of the phenotypic characteristics of Marfan's syndrome, such as familial thoracic aortic aneurysm or dissection, familial ectopia lentis and familial Marfan-like habitus.

The practical aims of treatment are to avoid contact sports and activities involving Valsalva's manoeuvre and anaerobic effort. Regular echocardiograms are used to pick up developing valvular prolapse/incompetence and to diagnose and arrange treatment of aneurysmal dilatation electively rather than as an emergency.

Ehlers–Danlos syndrome. Ehlers–Danlos syndrome covers a number of conditions, mostly inherited in an autosomal dominant pattern (but also recessive and sex-linked), characterized by abnormal soft connective tissue affecting the skin, tendons, ligaments and blood vessels. The result is joint laxity, easy bruising and skin fragility and hyperelasticity. The conditions have some overlap with other soft tissue problems associated with skin fragility and joint hypermobility, such as Marfan's syndrome and osteogenesis imperfecta. The conditions result from abnormalities of the fibrillar collagens type I, II, III and V. Abnormalities of type III are implicated in the most severe disease, which is characterized by death, often from arterial haemorrhage and colonic and uterine ruptures at the average age of 30 years.

Pseudoxanthoma elasticum. This is a rare autosomal recessive (but very occasionally autosomal dominant), progressive disease affecting the elastic tissues of the body. The incidence is between 1:25 000 and 1:50 000. The affected elastic fibres of the skin, eyes, heart and blood vessels are responsible for many of the symptoms associated with the condition. The skin becomes thickened, folded and discoloured. Calcification of blood vessels and hypertension lead to premature peripheral and coronary arterial disease, with an increased risk of mitral valve prolapse, and, in 50% of patients, angioid streaks are visible on fundoscopy. These are irregular, red–brown lines of variable width (from the barely visible to 3–4 times the diameter of the central retinal vein) radiating from the optic disc, which are also found in sickle cell anaemia and thalassaemia, Paget's disease of bone and certain pituitary disorders. Vision is frequently impaired by disciform degeneration of the central visual area.

Epidermolysis bullosa. This is a rare inherited disease of variable severity, characterized by the presence of a mutation of type VII collagen leading to extremely fragile skin. In severe cases, even touching the skin can cause painful blistering. Healing is often impaired and leads to scar formation and disfigurement. Blisters and scars in the gastrointestinal tract can cause malabsorption and blood loss, and predispose to infection.

Cutis laxa. This is a rare genetic connective tissue disorder usually transmitted in an autosomal recessive pattern, characterized by skin that lacks elasticity and therefore tends to hang loosely in wrinkles. The affected areas tend to be thickened and dark coloured.

MCQs

1 Marfan's syndrome is an autosomal recessive condition with a prevalence of 1:5000.
2 Marfan's syndrome typically involves the eye, the skeleton and the cardiovascular system.
3 In Marfan's syndrome, new mutations account for most of the cases seen.
4 Soft tissue sarcomas usually present with local pain.
5 Infection with human immunodeficiency virus predisposes to soft tissue sarcoma formation.

Case 6
Ear pain, deafness and a trivial nose bleed

History

A 48-year-old housewife presented to her GP complaining of progressive hearing loss, malaise, headaches and fevers, which were initially ascribed to recurrent middle ear infection and treated as such. Although the antibiotics did not produce much improvement, her symptoms were fairly stable, until a sneeze brought on an episode of acute severe pain in one ear for which she was seen in accident and emergency. She was admitted to hospital and, over the subsequent 36 h, became increasingly ill with deteriorating renal function and eventually anuria. The patient was transferred to the renal unit for haemodialysis, and high dose intravenous steroid treatment was instituted. A renal biopsy showed focal, segmental glomerulonephritis without granulomas. The patient and her husband explained that the patient had no history of epistaxis or haemoptysis at any time and that she had not suffered any significant illnesses in the past. Antineutrophil cytoplasmic antibodies (ANCAs) were positive.

Notes

The patient had developed Wegener's granulomatosis.

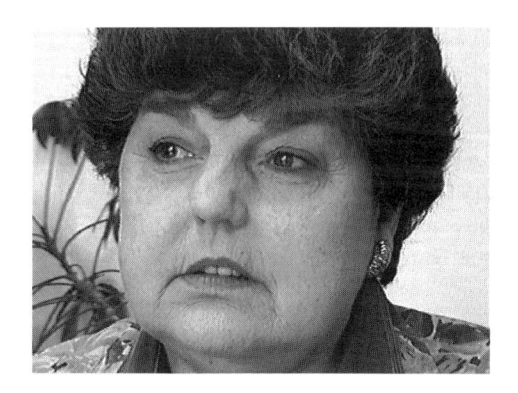

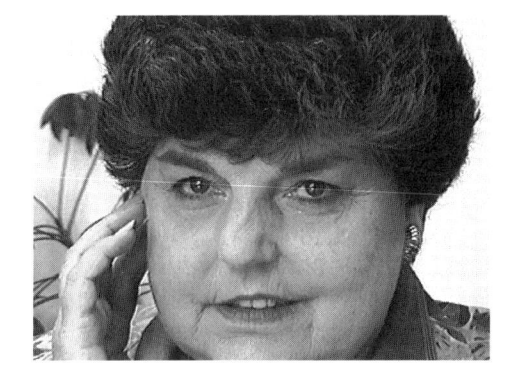

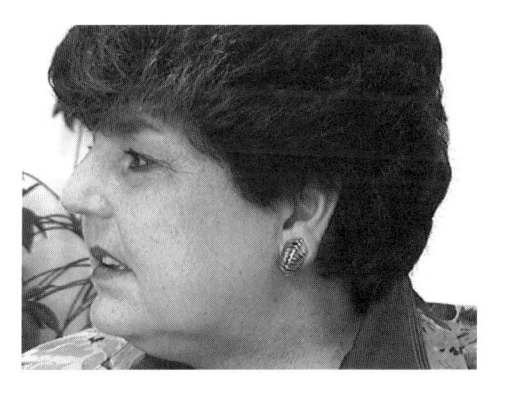

Wegener's granulomatosis is a necrotizing vasculitis associated with granuloma formation that classically affects the upper and lower respiratory tracts and nasopharynx in association with glomerulonephritis. Renal involvement, which often dominates the clinical picture, takes the form of focal, segmental glomerulitis with rapidly progressive crescentic glomerulonephritis (without granulomas). Typical presentations are with systemic features, such as pyrexia, malaise, arthralgias and weight loss, associated with a bloody nasal discharge due to mucosal ulceration that may progress to septal perforation. Blockage of the eustachian tube leads to otitis media, and pulmonary involvement, which occurs in most patients, manifests as cough, haemoptysis, dyspnoea and chest discomfort. The erythrocyte sedimentation rate (ESR) is usually markedly elevated, with hypergammaglobulinaemia, mild anaemia and leucocytosis. ANCAs are positive in 90% of cases and have a specificity of 80% (see 'Basic science').

Symptoms referred to the ear are unusual presenting manifestations of Wegener's granulomatosis. Bilateral corticosteroid-responsive sensorineural hearing loss and serous otitis media do occur however, and, particularly in young patients with Wegener's granulomatosis, organ involvement at presentation is often quite varied. Otalgia and otitis media or hearing loss, fulminant sinusitis, arthralgia and involvement of the oral cavity, skin, trachea and cornea, rather than classical rhinitis and nasal congestion, are all relatively common.

Basic science

Vasculitis

Vasculitis is inflammation and damage to blood vessels that may happen alone or as a component of another disease state. Vessels in any location may be affected, and the resulting changes often compromise blood flow and lead to ischaemia of the tissues supplied.

The deposition of immune complexes is widely accepted as the pathogenic mechanism involved, although direct evidence for this is usually absent. The deposition of immune complexes by platelets or mast cells into vasoactive amine-permeabilized vessels activates complement components which are chemotactic for neutrophils. These infiltrate the vessel wall, phagocytose the immune complexes and release enzymes that damage the vessel wall.

Other types of vasculitis

Polyarteritis nodosa. Polyarteritis nodosa is a multisystem necrotizing vasculitis of small- and medium-sized muscular arteries, typically affecting renal and visceral rather than pulmonary vessels. The mean age of onset is 45 years. Men are affected more than women, and the condition is characterized by weakness, headache, malaise, abdominal and muscle pain, often with prominent symptoms related to the organs predominantly involved. The involved vessels often have aneurysms up to 1 cm in diameter along their length. Hypertension and neutrophilia are common, a raised ESR is invariable, but eosinophilia is rare. About 30% of patients have glomerulitis and a similar proportion are hepatitis B surface antigen (HBsAg) positive.

Churg–Strauss disease. Churg–Strauss disease is a rare, necrotizing, granulomatous vasculitis (i.e. causes inflammation and destruction of blood vessels) similar in clinical manifestations to polyarteritis nodosa, but with a particular predilection to the lung and a strong association with late onset asthma and peripheral eosinophilia (of more than $1.5 \times 10^9\,L^{-1}$). Almost all patients with the condition have a history of asthma, and systemic vasculitis involving at least two extrapulmonary organs is a diagnostic prerequisite. Unlike other types of vasculitis, neurological involvement is common.

Temporal arteritis. Temporal arteritis, a panarteritis with mononuclear cell infiltrates of the vessel wall, occurs almost exclusively in those over 55 years of age. Patients are typically feverish, anorexic and have stiff, aching muscles with sweats, weight loss and headaches. Claudication of the tongue and jaw may occur, and ischaemic optic neuritis can rapidly cause blindness.

Takayasu's disease. Takayasu's disease is a vasculitic disease of unknown aetiology that occurs in the second or third decade of life. The panarteritis begins with adventitial inflammation and intimal proliferation, together with disruption and fibrotic changes in the media. Local pain is typically associated with involvement of the aortic arch vessels, and obliteration of the origins of the arch vessels with ischaemic retinopathy, blurred vision, syncope, dizziness, hypertension and absent pulses in the upper extremities are some of the symptoms and signs associated with this catastrophic condition.

Syphilis. Syphilis is essentially a disease of blood vessels. Fortunately, only 10% of those with syphilitic aortitis develop complications of saccular thoracic aneurysm, valvulitis and aortic regurgitation or coronary ostia stenosis during life.

Antineutrophil cytoplasmic antibodies (ANCAs)

The detection of circulating antibodies to neutrophil granule enzymes (ANCAs) is currently the only serological test for vasculitis. Unfortunately, although it is positive in 90% of patients with Wegener's granulomatosis, it is relatively non-specific, as it is also positive in infections and in inflammatory disease, as well as in autoimmune rheumatic diseases such as rheumatoid arthritis. ANCAs are positive in 70% of cases of idiopathic crescentic glomerulonephritis and 50% of cases of Churg–Strauss syndrome. A negative response is generally found in polyarteritis nodosa (10% positive only), Henoch–Schönlein purpura, Takayasu's disease and Kawasaki's disease. In human immunodeficiency virus disease, the significance of ANCA positivity (in up to 40% of cases) is doubtful.

In serum sickness, vasculitis is thought to result from the formation of immune complexes consisting of circulating antibodies and bacterial or viral proteins. In systemic lupus erythematosus (SLE), antibodies bind to cellular components and activate complement.

MCQs

1 Vasculitis is generally thought to be a degenerative process.
2 Polyarteritis nodosa typically affects the sinuses, nasopharynx, lower airways and kidneys.
3 ANCAs are positive in 50% of Wegener's granulomatosis.
4 Approximately 30% of patients with polyarteritis nodosa are HBsAg positive.
5 Churg–Strauss disease is strongly associated with late onset asthma.

Case 7
The woman with thigh pain and double vision

History

A 67-year-old housewife was admitted with a history of increasing pain in the left thigh over the previous month and a 10-day period of double vision particularly on looking to the right. Apart from some nausea associated with the diplopia, she claimed to feel well. She had a past history of rheumatic fever at the age of 15 years, and 30 years later had a Bjork Shiley (flap) aortic valve replacement. At the age of 58 years, a left mastectomy was performed for carcinoma of the breast.

On examination, the findings were in keeping with the thoracotomy and mastectomy described above. There were no visible abnormalities in her left thigh or leg, but extension and flexion of the thigh, which were not limited, increased the mid-thigh discomfort.

She was noted to have a right-sided abducent and partial right oculomotor nerve palsy. Her full blood count, urea, electrolytes and calcium were within normal limits. An isotope bone scan showed multiple hot spots.

Notes

The patient had multiple metastases from primary carcinoma of the breast.

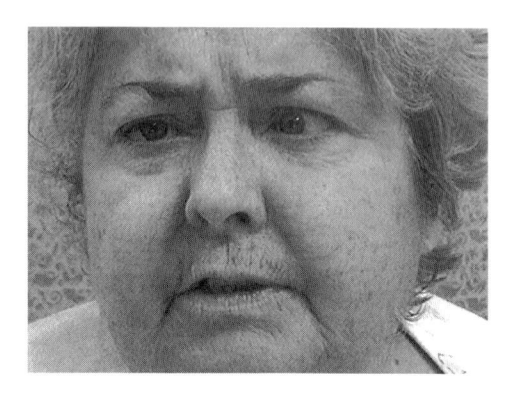

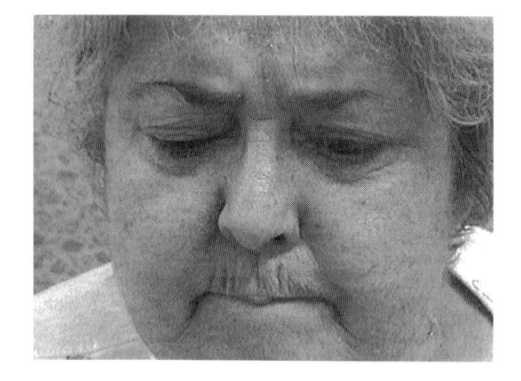

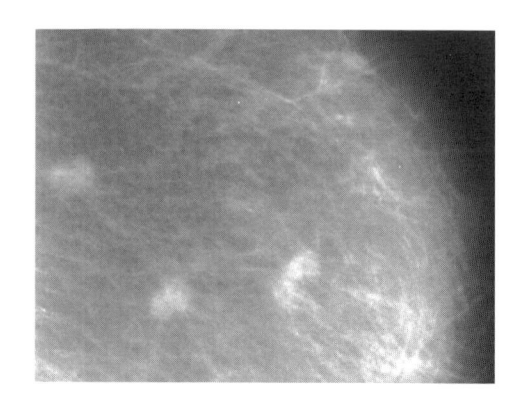

One in three people develop cancer during their lifetime and one in five die from it. With the exception of lung cancer, breast cancer is the most common neoplastic cause of death in women, with one woman in 11 contracting the disease. It is strongly related to lifetime oestrogen exposure and, like prostatic cancer, is highly responsive to endocrine manipulation. Risks are higher if a first order relative has the disease (particularly if it is the mother and she has bilateral disease), if menarche was early and if menopause was late. The risk of diagnosis of breast cancer (but not death from breast cancer) is higher in women who are concurrently taking female sex hormone replacement.

Breast cancer is usually multicentric at the time of diagnosis. This has been shown by the findings that at least 13% of patients with the disease have microscopic foci of tumour in other parts of the breast and that the incidence of occult intraductal carcinoma in women dying from unrelated causes after the age of 70 years is 19 times higher than the reported diagnosis rate *in vivo*. The size of the primary tumour, the number of axillary nodes involved in the disease, the presence of oestrogen receptors in tumour tissue and whether the patient is premenopausal or postmenopausal also have important prognostic significance. An oestrogen receptor-expressing tumour of less than 2 cm in diameter in a postmenopausal woman with no axillary nodal involvement is associated with the most favourable prognosis (over 80% 5-year survival). There is accumulating evidence that, in patients in whom bone marrow aspiration shows micrometastatic involvement, chronic treatment with bisphosphonates reduces the number of macroscopic metastases (in bone and other tissues) and increases survival.

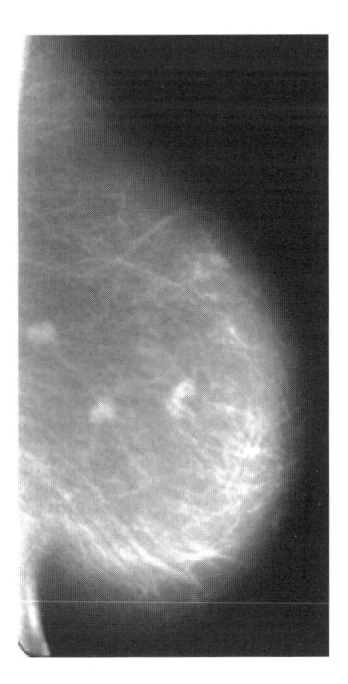

Basic science

Mechanisms of neoplasia

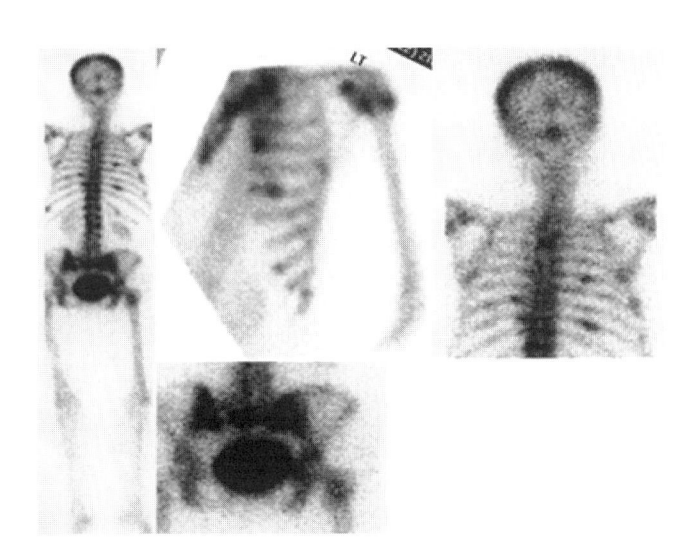

In almost all cases, cancer is thought to arise following malignant transformation of a single cell. In the clone of cells that results, in which proto-oncogenes have been activated or tumour suppressor genes inactivated or sequestered, growth is deregulated, normal function and differentiation are compromised and the capacity for dissemination is gained. Genetic factors and exposure to ultraviolet and ionizing radiation, tobacco smoke, asbestos and other organic and inorganic environmental mutagens, such as formaldehyde, benzene and alcohol, are implicated. There are also hereditary cancer syndromes, such as retinoblastoma, Gardner's syndrome (or polyposis coli), neurofibromatosis and the multiple endocrine neoplasia syndromes. Infections such as hepatitis B, which increases the incidence of hepatocellular carcinoma, Epstein–Barr virus, which is associated with Burkitt's lymphoma, and human immunodeficiency virus (HIV), which is associated with Kaposi's sarcoma and lymphomas of the central nervous system, are also strongly implicated in specific subtypes of neoplasia.

Tumour markers

- *Human chorionic gonadotrophin.* Normally made by placental trophoblast, and is made by trophoblastic tumours and germ cell tumours of the ovaries and testes.
- *Carcinoembryonic antigen.* Can be markedly elevated in cancers of the colon, pancreas, stomach, lung and breast.
- *α-Fetoprotein.* Produced by the gastrointestinal tract and liver during fetal development. Levels are raised in 70% of patients with hepatocellular carcinoma, testicular teratomas and occasionally in patients with gastrointestinal tumours.
- *Calcitonin levels.* Raised in patients with medullary carcinoma of the thyroid. Before genetic testing became available, calcitonin was used to diagnose the tumour in relatives of patients with multiple endocrine neoplasia types 2a and 2b.
- *Prostatic-specific antigen.* Raised in patients with carcinoma of the prostate and, to a lesser extent, in benign prostatic hypertrophy.
- *Monoclonal immunoglobulin bands.* Raised in multiple myeloma and monoclonal gammopathies.
- *Parathyroid hormone-related peptide (PTHRP).* This is a useful sign of a solid malignancy in the presence of hypercalcaemia.

MCQs

1 Breast cancer risk is strongly related to lifetime oestrogen exposure.
2 Breast tumours have a worse prognosis if they express oestrogen receptors.
3 Carcinoembryonic antigen is a tumour marker of germ cell tumours of the gonads.
4 α-Fetoprotein is raised in most cases of hepatocellular carcinoma.
5 In general, hypercalcaemia in malignancy is indicative of bone metastases.

Case 8
Lumps, bumps and palpitations

History

A 48-year-old postal clerk for a communications company was seen in clinic with a 1-month history of recurrent, fast palpitations. On each occasion, the onset of fast, regular palpitations would be quite sudden and the attacks would last for between 20 min and 1 h before gradually subsiding. The patient did not feel the need to pass urine after the attack, but felt quite tired afterwards. For the 2 days before she was seen, the patient had been more short of breath than usual, but denied any sweating or other physical or psychological symptoms during the attacks. Between attacks, the patient was very well, but had noticed that the lumps and bumps that had covered her body for as long as she could remember were getting more numerous. Her extraordinary back deformity had apparently remained stable for years.

Notes

The patient had developed a phaeochromocytoma complicating neurofibromatosis.

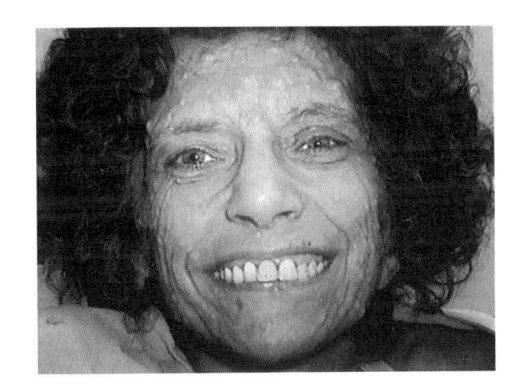

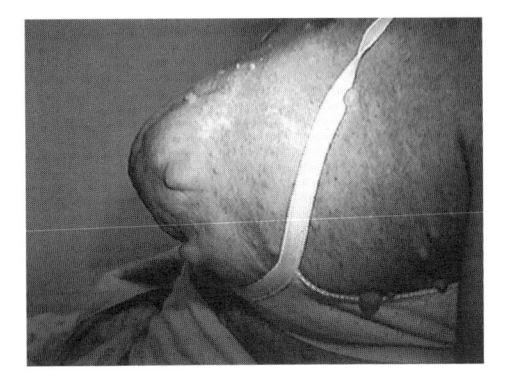

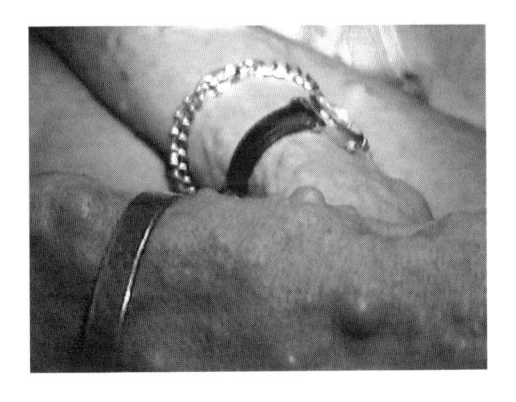

Neurofibromatosis (von Recklinghausen's syndrome) is one of a group of diseases, some of autosomal dominant heredity, that are characterized by neurological abnormalities and congenital defects of the skin, retina and other organs. Of this group of diseases, which include tuberous sclerosis (epiloia), ataxia telangiectasia, cerebelloretinal haemangioblastomatosis, Klippel–Trenaunay–Weber syndrome and Osler–Rendu–Weber syndrome, neurofibromatosis is by far the most common, with an incidence of 1:3000. In neurofibromatosis, multiple neurofibromas develop from the neurilemmal sheath of peripheral and cranial nerves. Patients are predisposed to intracranial neoplasms, such as gliomas, acoustic neuromas and meningiomas, and there is a rare association with phaeochromocytomas. The most common skin features are *café-au-lait* patches of skin pigmentation (typically more than five, each more than 2.5 cm in diameter), cutaneous fibromas and benign tumours of peripheral nerves, which appear as discrete, movable lumps arranged along lines of nerves.

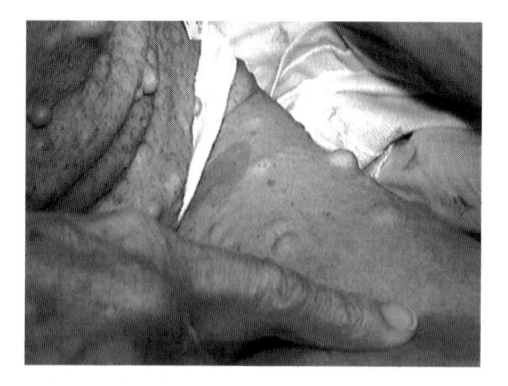

Basic science

Development of the neural crest

At the beginning of the third week of embryogenesis, the ectodermal germ layer begins to undergo the changes that transform it from a flat disc, the neural plate, into the central nervous system. The lateral edges of the neural plate increase in thickness to form neural folds either side of the neural groove and, as they do so, gradually come together in the midline. The first point of contact between the two neural folds is in the region of the future neck, from where fusion continues in cephalic and caudal directions to form the neural tube. The cephalic end of the neural tube closes over to separate it from the amniotic cavity at about day 25, and the caudal end closes soon after (day 27) to form a narrow tubular structure—the primitive spinal cord—supplanted by a much broader portion at the cephalic end. This bears the brain vesicles, several dilatations that give rise, respectively, to the forebrain (telencephalon and diencephalon, which in turn give rise to the cerebral hemispheres and the optic vesicles), the midbrain (mesencephalon) and the hindbrain (rhombencephalon), which later forms the pons, cerebellum and medulla oblongata. The cavities within the forebrain become the third ventricle and lateral ventricles, within the midbrain, the aqueduct of Sylvius, and within the hindbrain, the fourth ventricle.

Failure of closure of the distal spinal cord, spina bifida (myelomeningocoele), is the most common major birth defect amongst liveborn infants. A number of risk factors, such as maternal age, social class, heredity and birth order, have been identified for neural tube defects. More important is the recognition that the majority of neural tube defects can be prevented in the offspring of normal women by ensuring adequate intake of folate around the time of conception, and that, by reducing the number of antifolate drugs to a minimum and by introducing folate supplementation, the risk of neural tube defects in the offspring of women taking anticonvulsant drugs may be markedly reduced.

MCQs

1 The annual incidence of neurofibromatosis is ≈ 1 : 30 000.
2 The number of *café-au-lait* patches which suggests a diagnosis of neurofibromatosis is ≥5.
3 Patients with neurofibromatosis are predisposed to intracranial neoplasms.
4 In embryogenesis, the neural tube closes over in the second trimester of pregnancy.
5 The mesencephalon and rhombencephalon give rise to the structures of the brain stem.

Paradoxically, in some subtypes of lipodystrophy, a fatty liver can occur, and this can progress to cirrhosis and portal hypertension. This complication is unusual in the acquired partial form.

The diabetes mellitus that occurs with lipodystrophy behaves like typical non-insulin-dependent diabetes, but with higher levels of insulin resistance. Hypertriglyceridaemia may be accompanied by eruptive xanthomas, lipaemia retinalis and recurrent pancreatitis. Symptomatic coronary artery disease is rare. Hypermetabolism allows sufferers to ingest relatively large numbers of calories without gaining weight.

Other types of lipodystrophy include the following.
- *Dunnigan–Kobberling syndrome.* An autosomal dominant form of face-sparing partial lipodystrophy often associated with parental consanguinity.
- *Seip–Berardinelli syndrome.* This is characterized by lipodystrophy, hyperlipidaemia, hepatomegaly and insulin-resistant non-ketotic diabetes mellitus.
- *Cephalothoracic lipodystrophy.* This involves the face, arms and upper torso in association with mesangiocapillary glomerulonephritis.
- *Lawrence syndrome.* A sporadic type of generalized lipodystrophy with hepatomegaly, insulin-resistant diabetes mellitus and splenomegaly.

Basic science

Absorption of fat from the small intestines

Ingested fat is hydrolysed to monoacylglycerols and a smaller amount of glycerol and fatty acids in the intestinal lumen under the influence of pancreatic lipases. As these enzymes are water soluble, the fat must be converted from droplets which tend to coalesce into an emulsion in the duodenum to increase the surface area of reaction. With the aid of bile salts, the products of fat digestion are further reduced to micelles, 5 nm in diameter, which enter the intestinal wall where the monoacylglycerols are further broken down to free glycerol and fatty acids. The free glycerol formed within the intestinal lumen passes directly to the portal vein. The glycerol formed by hydrolysis of monoacylglycerols within the cells of the intestinal wall is reutilized directly for triglyceride synthesis and exported as chylomicrons and very low density lipoproteins (VLDLs) via the lymphatic system into the systemic circulation. The fat-soluble vitamins A (retinol) (used in the synthesis of visual pigments and to maintain epithelia), D (which facilitates the absorption of calcium and phosphate from the gut), E (antioxidant properties) and K (which facilitates the synthesis of clotting factors II, VII, IX and X) are absorbed with the fat. Under normal conditions, very little fat remains in the gut.

Hypertriglyceridaemia

The pathogenic role of hypertriglyceridaemia in coronary artery disease remains to be elucidated, but there is growing evidence that hypertriglyceridemia is a marker for several atherogenic factors and for increased risk of coronary artery disease. The atherogenic lipoprotein phenotype, or lipid triad, consists of elevated serum triglycerides, elevated levels of small low density lipoprotein (LDL) particles and low levels of high density lipoprotein (HDL) cholesterol. Hypertriglyceridaemia is also a marker for a metabolic syndrome in which the lipid changes noted above are associated with elevated blood pressure, insulin resistance and a prothrombotic state.

Causes of secondary hypertriglyceridaemia

- Diabetes.
- Alcohol abuse.
- Drugs (such as thiazide diuretics, β-blockers, retinoids, oral contraceptives).
- Obesity (with raised cholesterol).
- Renal disease (with raised cholesterol).
- Anorexia nervosa.

MCQs

1 The changes of lipodystrophy may not appear until after an attack of chicken pox.
2 Lipodystrophy is often associated with abnormalities of glucose and fat metabolism.
3 Lipodystrophy is often complicated by coronary heart disease.
4 Patients with lipodystrophy are often hypometabolic and tend to gain weight.
5 Isolated hypercholesterolaemia is a typical lipid profile in the lipodystrophies.

Case 20
Loss of libido, headaches and bad vision

History

A 20-year-old man was seen in clinic with an 8-year history of headaches which he described as being like an elastic band around the head. As he was otherwise well and had been progressing normally at school, the diagnoses of tension headaches or migraine were considered, and he and his family were reassured. The pains continued at intervals but, for the 6 months before he was seen in the outpatient department, he also complained of intermittent blurring of vision in the left eye, particularly when watching television, and visited the optician to see whether he needed glasses. The optician explained that he did not need glasses, but recommended that he see his GP with some urgency. He was referred from there to the outpatient department, where further symptoms of tiredness, lethargy and loss of libido were elicited. A formal visual field examination confirmed the presence of an upper temporal defect in his left eye and he was noted to have mild gynaecomastia. Fundoscopy and cranial nerve examination were otherwise unremarkable. His blood pressure was 112/76 mmHg.

Baseline blood tests revealed a testosterone level of $5.4\,nmol\,L^{-1}$ (normal range = $10–35\,nmol\,L^{-1}$), and the follicle-stimulating hormone (FSH) level was $3.6\,IU\,L^{-1}$ ($1–9\,IU\,L^{-1}$).

Notes

The patient had a macroprolactinoma pressing on his optic chiasm.

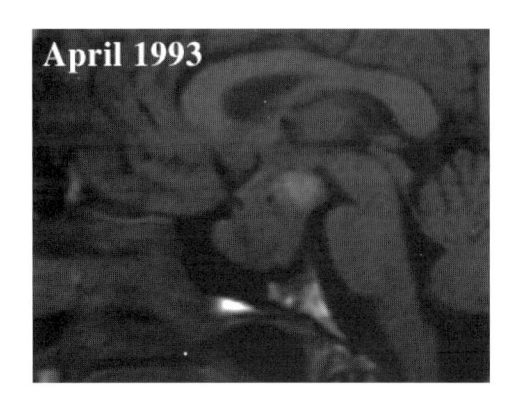

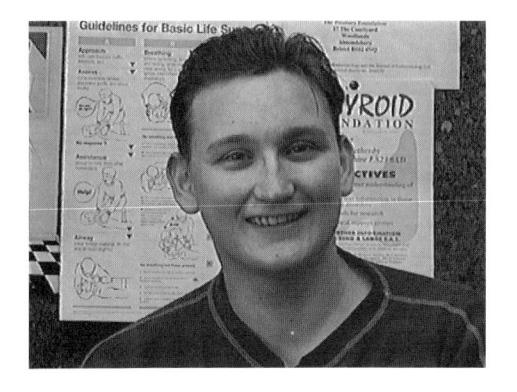

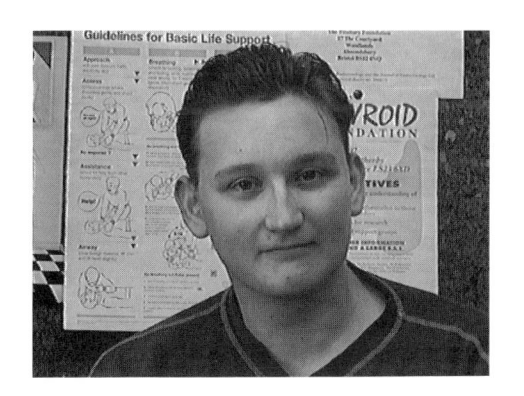

His prolactin, measured at the same time as gonadotrophins and sex hormones, was $34\,000\,mU\,L^{-1}$ (normal range = $\leq 800\,mU\,L^{-1}$). Prolactin is the anterior pituitary hormone responsible for inducing lactation in the oestrogen-primed breast. Raised levels of prolactin seen in the puerperium and, particularly during suckling-induced nipple stimulation, are associated with hypogonadotrophic hypogonadism (low oestrogen in association with low FSH and luteinizing hormone (LH) levels). For several weeks or sometimes months after delivery, libido and fertility are therefore reduced. Prolactin is a stress hormone, and modestly raised levels are seen after an epileptic fit or in stressful circumstances, such as in a patient who is particularly anxious about having a blood sample drawn. As hypothalamic dopamine is a prolactin release-inhibiting hormone, compression of the pituitary stalk by a non-secreting tumour or treatment with dopamine antagonists, such as metoclopramide, phenothiazines or domperidone, can cause hyperprolactinaemia. Some cases of polycystic ovarian disease are also associated with mild hyperprolactinaemia. The most common pathological cause of a raised prolactin level is the presence of a microprolactinoma, a prolactin-secreting pituitary adenoma of less than 10 mm in diameter contained within the sella turcica. Prolactin levels in excess of $15\,000\,mUL^{-1}$ are usually due to macroprolactinomas. Both micro- and macroprolactinomas are usually highly responsive to treatment with dopamine agonists.

Basic science

Breast development

The male and female breasts are identical until puberty. At this time, an increase in circulating oestrogens from the ovary stimulates breast ductal development and the local deposition of fat and connective tissue. The first sign of this is development of the breast bud, a small pad of sometimes slightly tender tissue beneath the nipple and areolae. Each successive cycle of oestrogen formation from the granulosa cells surrounding developing ovarian follicles stimulates further breast development.

During pregnancy, the placenta produces very large quantities of oestrogen and progesterone which, in the presence of prolactin, stimulate further breast ductal and lobuloalveolar growth. Delivery of the placenta at the third stage of labour results in a dramatic fall in oestrogen and progesterone, leaving prolactin free to induce lactation in the oestrogen-primed breast. Once lactation is established, a month or two after delivery, oxytocin release in anticipation of nursing, together with suckling-induced increases in prolactin and oxytocin, maintain lactation even when prolactin levels between nursing episodes return to well within normal values.

High levels of prolactin are rarely enough to induce lactation in a man as, under normal circumstances, male breasts have not been oestrogen primed.

Gynaecomastia

Gynaecomastia, the presence of palpable breast tissue, is found in 40% of normal men and is considered physiological in neonates, during puberty and in old age when the ambient oestrogen/androgen ratio is relatively high.

Differential diagnosis of gynaecomastia

- Idiopathic.
- Deficient androgen production:
    Klinefelter's syndrome.
    Secondary testicular failure (orchitis, trauma, castration, renal failure).
    Androgen resistance syndromes (such as testicular feminization).
- Increased oestrogen production:
    Testicular tumours (often rapidly developing, painful gynaecomastia).
    Carcinoma of the lung producing oestrogens.
    Increased substrate for peripheral aromatase (starvation (particularly on refeeding), thyrotoxicosis, adrenal disease, liver disease and the use of very high levels of anabolic androgens by bodybuilders and athletes).

- Drugs:
  Gonadotrophin-releasing hormone superagonists and antiandrogens, such as finasteride and flutamide (used in prostatic disease). Digoxin, spironolactone, cimetidine and ketoconazole also inhibit testosterone synthesis, and marijuana and heroin are associated with gynaecomastia through unknown mechanisms.

MCQs

1 Large amounts of oestrogen, progesterone and prolactin are produced by the placenta.
2 Very high levels of prolactin in men commonly cause galactorrhoea.
3 Prolactin levels of over 15 000 mU L^{-1} (≤800 mU L^{-1}) are invariably caused by macroprolactinomas.
4 Prolactin levels are increased by suckling.
5 Unilateral visual field problems are rare in pituitary tumours.

Case 21
As smooth as a baby's bottom

History

A 65-year-old retired shopkeeper was seen in the outpatient department with a history of erectile dysfunction stretching back more than 10 years. He was not too concerned about this because his libido was minimal. Tiredness was a problem, however, and he claimed that lethargy was at times so overwhelming that, even after a full night's sleep, he could return to bed after breakfast and sleep for several hours more. On direct questioning, he explained that he shaved his beard twice a week and that, having never been 'a particularly hairy person', his skin was now 'as smooth as a baby's bottom'.

On examination, he was noted to have fine, pale skin with no chest, axillary or pubic hair. His testes were small and soft, and his blood pressure was 134/72 mmHg with no postural drop. Visual fields were full to confrontation.

Notes

The patient had primary hypopituitarism.

The most likely cause in this case was autoimmune destruction of the anterior pituitary. The diagnosis was confirmed biochemically as the patient's circulating testosterone level was 2.6 nmol L^{-1} (normal range = 10–25 nmol L^{-1}), with levels of follicle-stimulating hormone (FSH) of 3 IU L^{-1} (1–9 IU L^{-1}), luteinizing hormone (LH) of 3 IU L^{-1} (3–8 IU L^{-1}), free thyroxine of 10 pmol L^{-1} (10–23 pmol L^{-1}), thyroid-stimulating hormone (TSH) of 0.5 mU L^{-1} (0.3–6 mU L^{-1}), prolactin of 140 mU L^{-1} (<800 mU L^{-1}) and random cortisol of 185 nmol L^{-1} (150–800 nmol L^{-1}). A Synacthen test showed a rise in cortisol to 300 nmol L^{-1} over 1 h (normal response >495 nmol L^{-1}). A magnetic resonance scan of his pituitary was unremarkable.

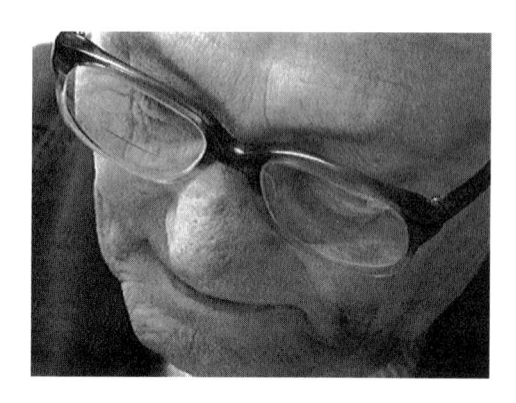

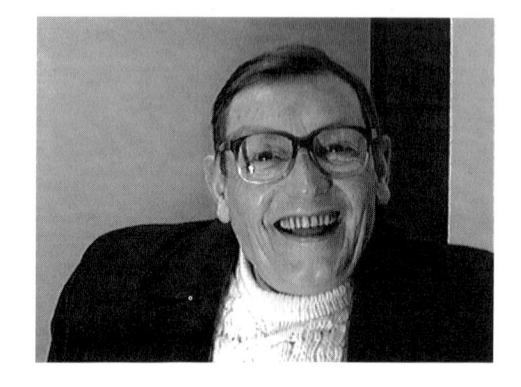

Most cases seen in clinic are related to endocrinologically inactive pituitary adenomas compressing the normal pituitary or to surgery or radiotherapy for pituitary tumours or craniopharyngiomas.

The symptoms and signs experienced by this patient are caused by a combination of slowly progressive secondary hypogonadism, hypoadrenalism and hypothyroidism. The reduction in circulating hormones, which is more modest than would be seen in primary endocrine gland failure, is very typical.

Differential diagnosis of hypogonadotrophic hypogonadism

- Hypothalamic tumours:
    Craniopharyngiomas.
    Dysgerminomas.
    Hamartomas.
- Prolactinomas.
- Granulomatous and infiltrative disorders:
    Langerhans cell histiocytosis.
    Cerebral sarcoidosis.
- Parasellar lesions:
    Meningiomas.
    Optic nerve tumours.

Basic science

Immune system-mediated diseases can be divided into the following:
- Immunodeficiency, in which either the absence or inactivity of components of the immune system predisposes an individual to infection with particular pathogens.
- Hypersensitivity, in which the target of the immune attack is appropriate, but the response is out of proportion to the threat it poses.
- Autoimmunity, in which the immune system recognizes and reacts against the body's own tissues. Exposure of the developing immune system to antigens during fetal or early postnatal life results in the deletion of self-reactive clones through mechanisms that are not clearly understood. The development of autoreactive clones in later life is also very complex and involves multiple genes and environmental events, such as infection and drug treatment.

Autoimmune diseases are produced by deregulated T-cell control of the immune system, leading to the generation of autoreactive T cells or to the production of host tissue-reactive antibodies. Typical examples are autoimmune thyrotoxicosis (Graves' disease) or hypothyroidism (Hashimoto's disease), insulin-dependent diabetes mellitus, myasthenia gravis, autoimmune adrenal failure (Addison's disease) and the spectrum of antibodies to DNA, platelets and red cells that occurs in systemic lupus erythematosus. Recent studies suggest that, in some patients, there is excessive programmed cell death following viral illnesses or in response to environmental stimuli. This may be associated with inappropriate exposure of autoantigens to the immune system.

MCQs

1 Hypothyroidism secondary to pituitary failure is often more mild than primary hypothyroidism.
2 Exposure of the immune system to antigens during fetal or early postnatal life results in tolerance.
3 In hypopituitarism, the skin is usually smooth and pale.
4 TSH, FSH and LH levels within the normal range exclude hypopituitarism.
5 B lymphocytes kill human cells displaying foreign antigens, such as virus proteins.

Case 22
The perils of a 'lie in'

History

A 32-year-old man was admitted following a *grand mal* convulsion. His first episode of loss of consciousness was witnessed by his partner with whom he had been building a dry stone wall, 15 years previously. He remembers 'feeling funny' while carrying a pail of water back to the wall from an adjacent field, and the next thing he knew he was in an ambulance. In hospital, he was told that 'every young adult was allowed a single fit' and that they would not investigate him further unless the problem recurred. It did not recur for 15 years, but then occurred twice in quick succession, once while cycling and the second time within seconds of getting out of a swimming pool. Subsequently, the attacks began to happen more frequently, and he began to recognize the visual aura—the appearance of a white spot in his field of vision—and other feelings that preceded them. His partner noticed that he would become vague and sweat excessively at the beginning of an attack, and that the attacks were related to exercise, exacerbated by 'having a lie in' (which entailed a late breakfast) and relieved by eating, provided that he was able to do so quickly enough. As a result, he had noted a 32 lb increase in weight over the previous 6 months.

Notes

The patient had developed an insulinoma.

The relationship to food, increase in weight, sweating and other symptoms of neuroglycopenia (low cerebral blood glucose) were noted and the patient was given home blood glucose monitoring apparatus on which he recorded levels of 1.2 mmol L^{-1} during a number of attacks. Pancreatic angiography

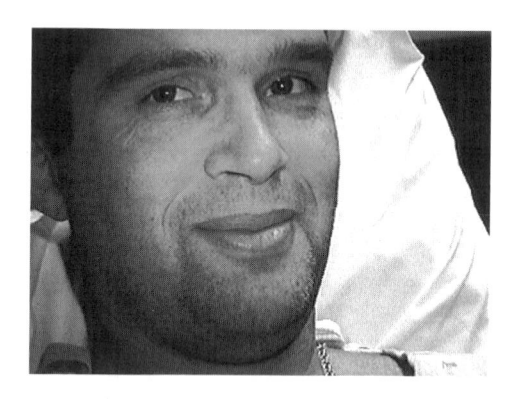

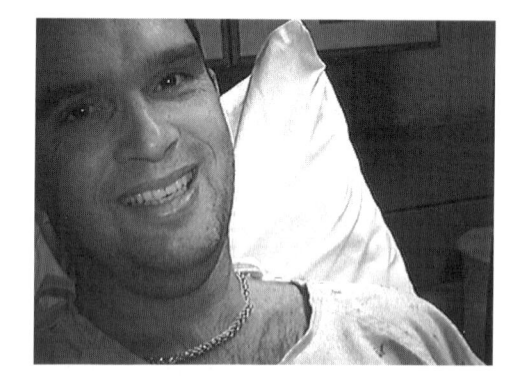

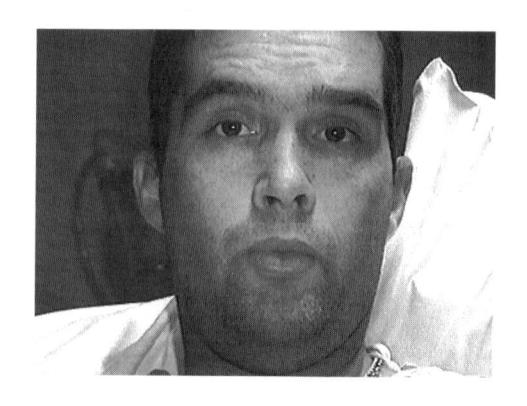

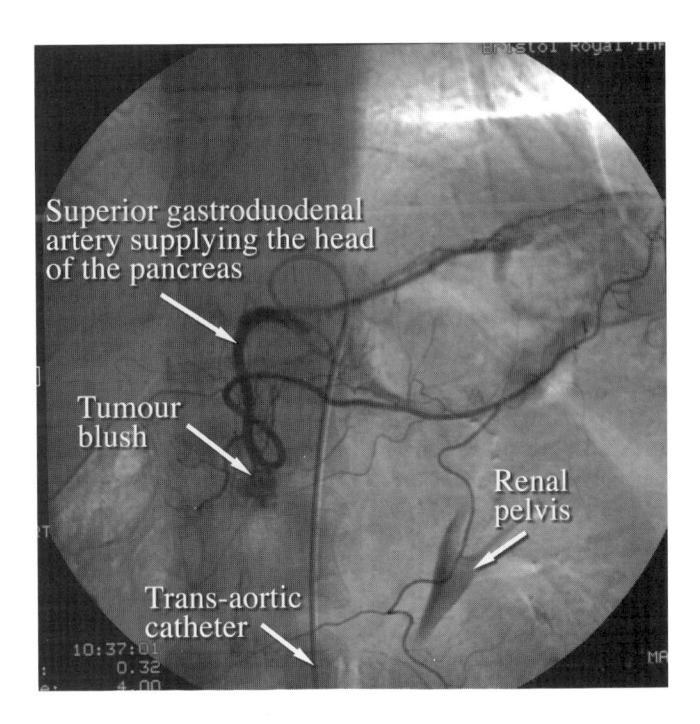

![Angiogram with labels: Superior gastroduodenal artery supplying the head of the pancreas; Tumour blush; Renal pelvis; Trans-aortic catheter]

was carried out and, to further define the location of the lesion, right hepatic venous blood samples were collected before and at 30, 60, 90, 120 and 180 s after a bolus infusion of calcium gluconate (2.5 mg kg^{-1} body weight) into each of the four vascular territories of the pancreas. A dramatic increase in insulin secretion from the involved territory confirmed the localization of the lesion.

Insulinomas are rare endocrine tumours with an estimated incidence of 1:1 000 000. Optimal therapy is surgical resection and, if the biochemical diagnosis can be made with considerable certainty, the 40% of tumours that are not identifiable by computerized tomography (CT) scan, by transabdominal ultrasound or by angiography can usually be detected without problems between the palpating fingers of an experienced surgeon. As even the presence of a 'tumour blush' on contrast angiography can be misleading, injections of calcium gluconate as an insulin secretogogue into the proximal gastroduodenal, proximal splenic, inferior pancreaticoduodenal, proper hepatic and superior mesenteric arteries can be carried out in turn, with sampling in the right hepatic vein close to its junction with the inferior vena cava.

Basic science

Insulin is a polypeptide hormone consisting of an α and a β chain, synthesized and secreted from the β cells of the pancreatic islets of Langerhans. Proinsulin, the precursor protein, is cleaved into mature insulin and 'C peptide', which can be used as a biochemical marker of endogenous insulin secretion. Under normal circumstances, unless a large bolus of glucose is ingested, the rapid insulin secretory response of the pancreas (within 60 s from the limited stores—followed by a more sustained release of newly synthesized peptide) is enough to ensure that circulating glucose concentrations vary little. About half of the insulin secreted from the pancreas is inactivated by first pass metabolism in the liver, which itself is an important target organ for insulin action.

The principal metabolic effects of insulin on

most cells (with the exception of those of the brain and liver) are to increase the uptake of glucose and amino acids, and stimulate glycogen, fat and protein synthesis.

Glucagon and other hormones, such as epinephrine and growth hormone, have effects that essentially oppose those of insulin. After a high carbohydrate meal, insulin levels rise in response to increasing glucose levels and glucagon secretion from the α cells of the pancreatic islets is depressed. After a protein meal, circulating amino acid levels increase without a corresponding increase in glucose. Insulin levels rise, but, if unopposed, would cause hypoglycaemia. A concurrent rise in glucagon prevents this by mediating hepatic gluconeogenesis and glycogenolysis.

Hypoglycaemic coma caused by an accidental overdose of exogenous insulin can be reversed by an intramuscular injection of 1 mg glucagon. Once the patient has recovered consciousness, he/she can be given glucose or another readily absorbable carbohydrate orally.

MCQs

1 Insulin and C peptide are produced by the pancreas in equimolar amounts.
2 Most patients who present with 'funny feelings relieved by eating' harbour insulinomas.
3 All of the insulin secreted by the pancreas reaches the systemic circulation unchanged.
4 An intramuscular injection of glucagon is a useful treatment in hypoglycaemic coma.
5 Patients with insulinomas tend to be thin.

Case 23
The man who couldn't mount a camel

History

A 63-year-old business consultant was seen in clinic with erectile dysfunction and modest short-term memory impairment. He was otherwise well, but alleged that his upper body strength had always been poor. Puberty had taken place at a normal time and was, as far as he could recall, uneventful. His muscular development had increased little, however, and it had never been easy for him, for example, to raise weights above his head. In his early twenties, he married and, after a number of years of sexual intercourse which failed to result in his partner's pregnancy, he was investigated for infertility. The tests carried out at the time failed to identify a cause, and it was not until he was 40 years old that further investigations, including a testicular biopsy, were carried out and the diagnosis was made.

Notes

The patient had Klinefelter's syndrome.

Testicular biopsy showed hyalinization of the seminiferous tubules and azoospermia, features consistent with a diagnosis of Klinefelter's syndrome.

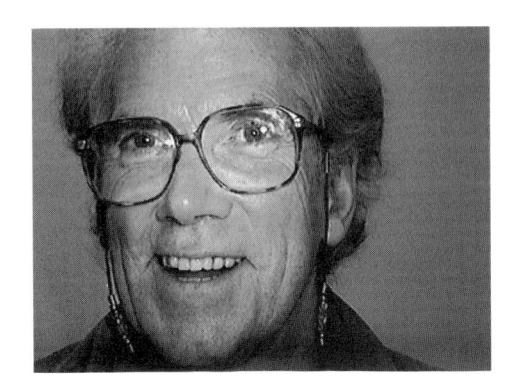

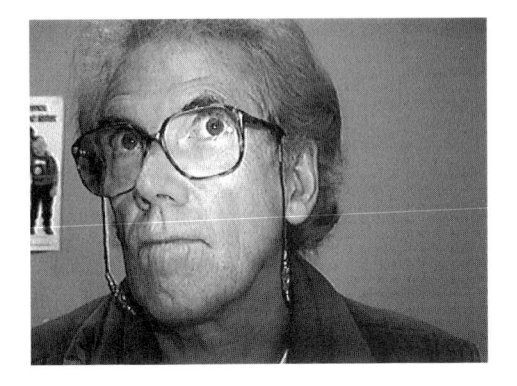

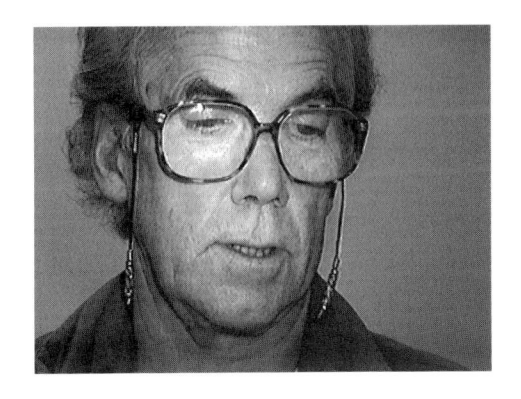

Klinefelter's syndrome, most commonly caused by the 47,XXY genotype, is the most common chromosomal cause of abnormal sexual differentiation. In 10% of cases, the patient is a 46,XY/47,XXY mosaic, and many additional phenotypes with increasing numbers of X chromosomes in pure or mosaic form have also been described. In some of these, the mosaicism is only present in the testes (which may be of normal size) and will therefore be missed on routine peripheral white blood cell karyotype analysis. The 47,XXY phenotype is characterized by small, firm testes (contrasting with the small, soft testes characteristic of alcoholism), oligospermia or azoospermia and elevated levels of gonadotrophins (luteinizing hormone (LH) and follicle-stimulating hormone (FSH)) consistent with primary hypogonadism. Gynaecomastia, which can be marked, is associated with an increased risk of breast cancer. Other symptoms and signs of hypoandrogenaemia, tall stature and mild mental deficiency are also variable features. Internal and external genitalia and psychosexual orientation are male.

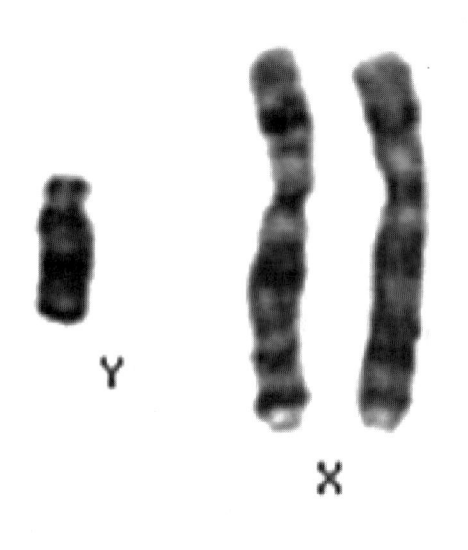

Basic science

The normal human genome consists of 23 pairs of chromosomes (22 somatic and 1 sex). These are duplicated prior to mitosis and returned to the normal diploid complement by cell division. In meiosis, two consecutive cell divisions are required. Prior to the first division, the chromosomes are duplicated and line up in homologous pairs in the equatorial plane of the cell by attachment of the centromere to the spindle as in mitosis. In meiosis, however, the duplicated chromosomes remain attached at their centromeres and the process of 'crossing over' occurs. In this process, chromosomes break at identical points along their length, and subsequently rejoin before they are drawn apart to opposite poles of the cell. After division, the two cells contain only one duplicated copy of each chromosome, held together at the centromeres. In the second meiotic division, the sister chromatids, previously held together at the centromeres, separate to yield four haploid cells (i.e. containing only one copy of each chromosome) known as gametes.

Stable, heritable alterations in DNA are known as mutations. Chromosomal deletions (loss of a section of the chromosome), translocations (transfer of sections of a chromosome to an ectopic genomic site) and duplications (such as trisomy 21, giving rise to Down's syndrome) are often visible on light microscopic examination of the chromosomes (karyotype analysis). Other mutations, such as substitution of a single base pair for another (point mutation), cannot be seen directly, but will change the codon in which they occur. Deletions and insertions move the codon reading frame (frame shift mutations) and result in the formation of a nonsense protein or, more usually, no detectable protein at all. Single base substitutions give rise to conditions such as sickle cell anaemia.

MCQs

1 The 47,XXY genotype is not universal in Klinefelter's syndrome.
2 The genotypic abnormality of Klinefelter's syndrome may be confined to testicular tissue.
3 Patients with Klinefelter's syndrome have an increased risk of testicular cancer.
4 In Klinefelter's syndrome, gonadotrophin (FSH and LH) levels are usually low.
5 In meiosis as opposed to mitosis, chromosomal duplication does not occur.

Case 24
Spousal arousal

History

A 44-year-old man was first seen in clinic at the age of 24 years. He had only been married for a short time when his wife complained that he was keeping her awake by involuntarily rubbing his arms during the night. The patient acknowledged that he had woken from sleep at intervals for years with aching forearms and wrists, but it was only when his new wife insisted that he seek help that he presented to his GP.

He had been a physically very active man in his youth who, during his teenage years, graduated from sailing dinghies to full ocean racing. He had assumed that the large size of his hands was partly the result of his job as a winch hand and, indeed, he was one of the few crew members who was able to operate the machinery single handed. Standing 6 ft 4.5 in (194 cm) in his stockinged feet, he explained that, between the ages of 9 and 13 years, he grew more than 1 ft (30.5 cm) in height rather than the average increase of just over half that amount (16.5 cm).

Notes

The patient had gigantism, an extremely rare condition that results from the development of a growth hormone-secreting somatotrophic adenoma of the pituitary prior to puberty.

The condition persisted through puberty and beyond, but because the tumour did not render him hypogonadotrophic (i.e. at least partially hypopituitary), he progressed through puberty and fused his epiphyses at an appropriate age, preventing further inappropriate linear growth.

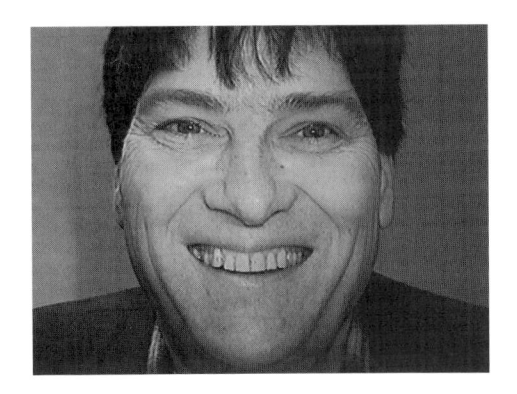

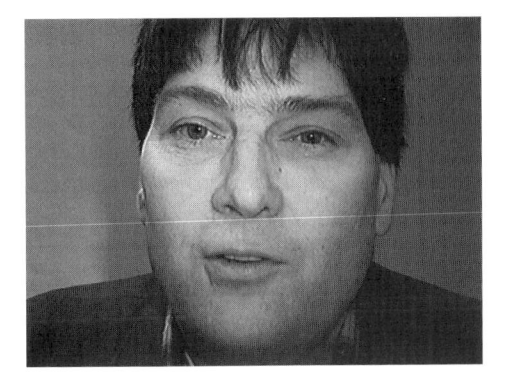

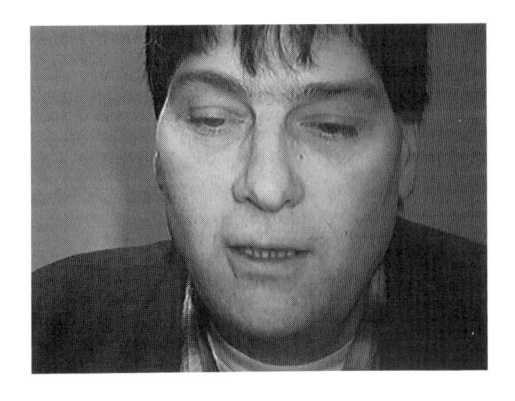

The diagnosis made by the GP was acromegaly, and this was confirmed by CT scan of his pituitary fossa and raised circulating growth hormone levels which increased in response to an oral glucose load (instead of decreasing) and increased (also paradoxically) in response to thyrotrophin-releasing hormone. He was treated successfully with transphenoidal adenomectomy.

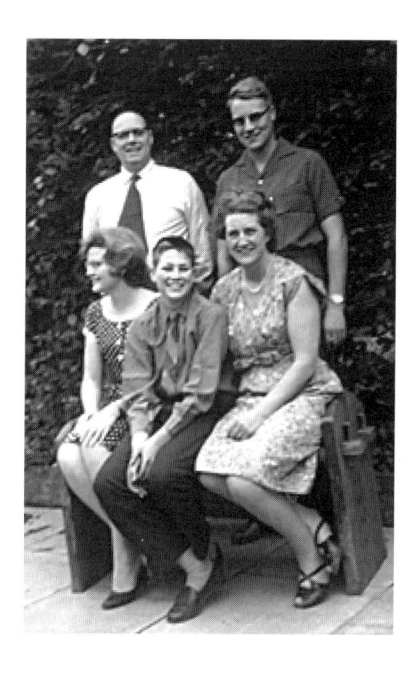

Basic science

Stature

Growth in the first year after birth is extremely rapid, with a doubling in weight and a 50% increase in body length. An individual's growth throughout childhood from the age of 2 years until puberty tends to follow a percentile channel of a growth chart with remarkable stability, provided that it is derived from an up to date analysis of an appropriate population. Boys enter puberty at an average age of 11.5 years, 8 months later than girls on average, and the more prolonged period of prepubertal growth that this allows, together with a more intensive pubertal growth spurt, accounts for the greater mean adult height in men.

Growth hormone deficiency as a cause of short stature is unusual, the more usual causes being:
- short parents (who may be normal-short or may have passed on a treatable cause of short stature),
- poor nutrition,
- social or emotional deprivation,
- intrauterine growth retardation, or
- poorly treated chronic medical conditions, such as coeliac disease, asthma, colitis or renal failure.

The hormonal control of growth is complex and not well understood. A useful model is that, during childhood and adolescence, limb growth is mediated predominantly by growth hormone and spinal growth by sex hormones. A long period of prepubertal growth in a male who enters puberty (and is therefore exposed to androgens) relatively late results in a eunuchoid habitus, characterized by long legs and a relatively short body. An early puberty, in contrast, tends to fuse epiphyses of long bones early and encourages axial/spinal growth, resulting in short legs supplanted by a long body.

There are as many cases of constitutional tall stature as there are short, but, as the same social stigma does not apply, their presentation is unusual unless accompanied by other problems. Gigantism, the condition described above, is extremely rare. Tall stature is more usually associated with tall parents, Klinefelter's syndrome (XXY) and XYY males, thyrotoxicosis, Marfan's syndrome and homocystinuria. Tall, fat children are almost always the product of chronic overnutrition throughout childhood.

MCQs

1 Some patients with gigantism can continue to grow in height throughout their lives.
2 During the first year of life, weight usually doubles and length increases by 50%.

3 Boys enter puberty on average 8 months later than girls.
4 Limb and spinal linear growth is mediated by growth hormone.
5 An individual's adult height can normally be predicted at the age of 2 years.

Case 25
A smaller cup of coffee

History

A 36-year-old sales manager was seen in clinic with a 6-month history of progressive weakness. She had always been overweight and, apart from backaches which she assumed were a consequence of the same, had always considered herself fit and well. In retrospect, however, over the preceding 6 months, she had found it more difficult to stand up after sitting on the floor, and the increasing strain of holding a kettle under the tap was resulting in her putting less and less water in it to boil. Her skin had not changed in appearance, but she felt that she bruised more easily than normal and that, although always 'big', she had put on over 30 lb in weight over the previous few months.

On examination, the patient was centrally obese and, aside from moderate facial hirsutism, her skin appeared normal, with no thinning, bruising or striae. Her blood pressure was 146/86 mmHg.

Notes

The patient had Cushing's disease (pituitary-dependent Cushing's syndrome).

The diagnosis was confirmed biochemically with two 24-h collections of urine for cortisol and creatinine (to ensure a complete collection) which showed levels of 960 and 1230 nmol per 24 h (normal range <275 nmol per 24 h). After a single 1 mg tablet of dexamethasone taken at 11 p.m., the patient's 9 a.m. cortisol level was suppressed to 200 nmol L^{-1} (≤138 nmol L^{-1}) from a baseline cortisol measured on two occasions of between 750 and 830 nmol L^{-1}. Her adrenocorticotrophic hormone (ACTH) level was modestly elevated at 43 ng L^{-1} (normal range 5–36 at 9 a.m.) (at 9 a.m.). A magnetic resonance imaging (MRI) scan showed a small, hypodense area in a pituitary gland of essentially normal size.

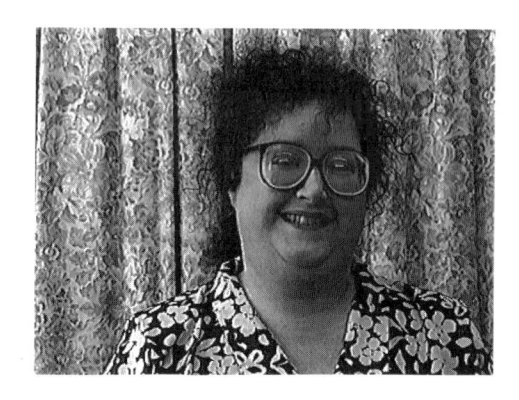

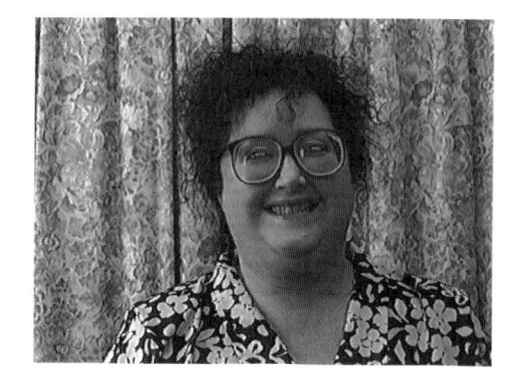

Cushing's disease is a classical, but rare, endocrine disease. It is characterized symptomatically by mental changes (often accentuation of premorbid personality), weight gain, proximal myopathy (difficulty standing from sitting without using the arms), muscle wasting, central accumulation of fat (filling in the temporal fossae and producing the characteristic 'moon face' and 'buffalo hump'), weakening of the skin leading to the formation of wide, purple stretch marks (striae) and easy bruisability. Hypertension, hirsutism (due to increased ACTH drive to adrenal androgen production) and glucose intolerance are also common. In Cushing's disease, the ACTH-induced increase in the production of adrenal preandrogens (responsible for hirsutism) tends to protect against steroid-induced thinning of the skin.

Basic science

Glucocorticoids

Glucocorticoids diffuse into their target cells, combine with cytoplasmic receptor protein and are transported to the nucleus where they modify gene expression and protein synthesis.

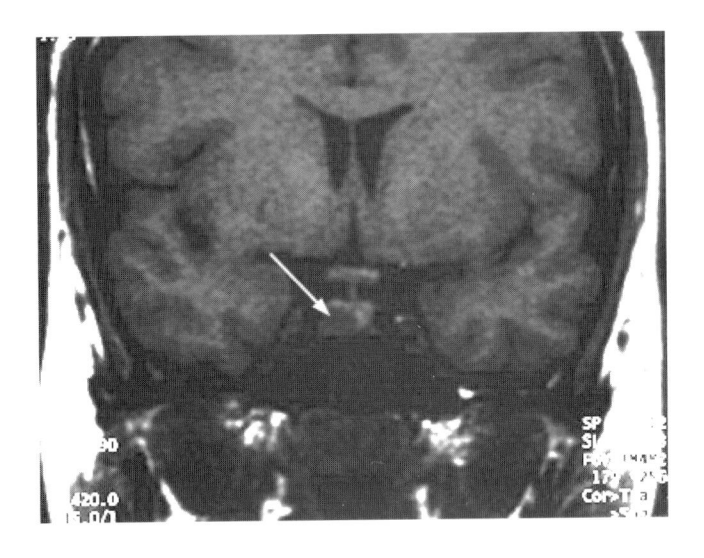

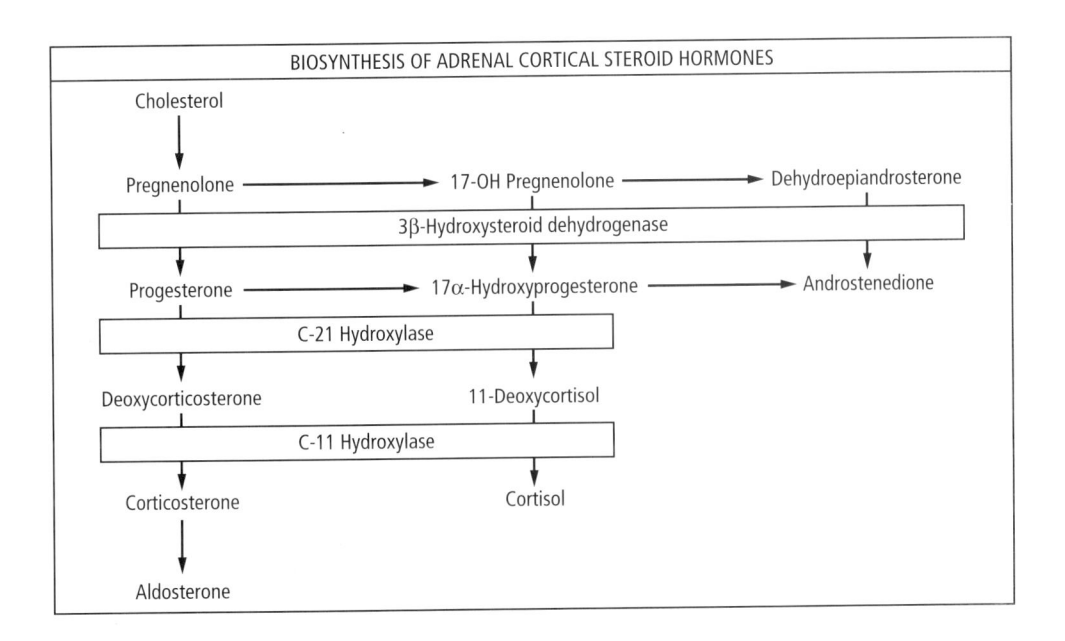

```
BIOSYNTHESIS OF ADRENAL CORTICAL STEROID HORMONES

Cholesterol
    ↓
Pregnenolone ─────────→ 17-OH Pregnenolone ─────────→ Dehydroepiandrosterone
                    3β-Hydroxysteroid dehydrogenase
    ↓                            ↓                              ↓
Progesterone ─────────→ 17α-Hydroxyprogesterone ─────────→ Androstenedione
                           C-21 Hydroxylase
    ↓                            ↓
Deoxycorticosterone       11-Deoxycortisol
                           C-11 Hydroxylase
    ↓                            ↓
Corticosterone              Cortisol
    ↓
Aldosterone
```

They have many effects on metabolism, including stimulation of hepatic glucose synthesis, breakdown of protein in muscle, skin and bone, an anti-inflammatory effect and enhancement of lipid mobilization. In addition to their immune effects and effects on carbohydrate, protein and fat metabolism, glucocorticoids also have profound effects on salt and water metabolism, causing marked sodium retention and potassium loss. Cortisol, the principal circulating glucocorticoid, protects us from stress-induced hypotension, shock and death by mechanisms that are not understood.

Only 1% of cortisol is excreted in the urine unchanged. Most undergoes hepatic metabolism by reduction, oxidation, hydroxylation and conjugation reactions.

Glucocorticoid synthesis

Glucocorticoids are synthesized from cholesterol by enzymes in the adrenal cortex. Syndromes caused by inherited defects in the enzymatic synthesis of cortisol are rather misleadingly called congenital adrenal hyperplasia. A common feature of the condition is that negative feedback of cortisol on the pituitary is diminished, and pituitary ACTH secretion is increased. Clinical manifestations combine excessive production of precursor steroids, including 17-hydroxyprogesterone, which is often exploited as a biochemical marker, and androgens. In some subtypes, aldosterone production is also decreased.

MCQs

1 Thinning of the skin is one of the most useful clinical signs of Cushing's disease (i.e. pituitary-dependent Cushing's syndrome).
2 Cortisol is largely excreted unchanged.
3 In congenital adrenal hyperplasia, the adrenals are large from birth.
4 Proximal myopathy is a useful sign to distinguish obesity from Cushing's syndrome.
5 17-Hydroxyprogesterone is increased in congenital adrenal hyperplasia.

Case 26
Nasal discharge

History

A 55-year-old businessman visited his optician complaining that a dark image seemed to be present at the edge of his vision. The optician excluded a detached retina and refractory defects, but identified marked, bilateral upper temporal quadrant field loss. He was referred to hospital but, before the appointment date, suddenly developed a severe headache and collapsed. An urgent magnetic resonance imaging (MRI) scan showed a pituitary macroadenoma with surrounding blood in the subarachnoid space. A diagnosis of pituitary apoplexy was made and, after a 24-h period of stabilization, he had a successful and uneventful transphenoidal adenomectomy which revealed haemorrhagic fragments of an endocrinologically inactive pituitary adenoma. He was seen in the outpatient department 3 weeks later and explained that, soon after returning home, he had noticed a salty taste in the back of his mouth and, if he leant forward, clear fluid would drip from his nose. Much to his surprise, he was immediately readmitted to hospital.

Notes

The patient had a persistent cerebrospinal fluid (CSF) leak through the bony deficit made in the floor of his pituitary fossa. Its presence is an urgent indication for corrective surgery, and he was readmitted so that the defect could be patched.

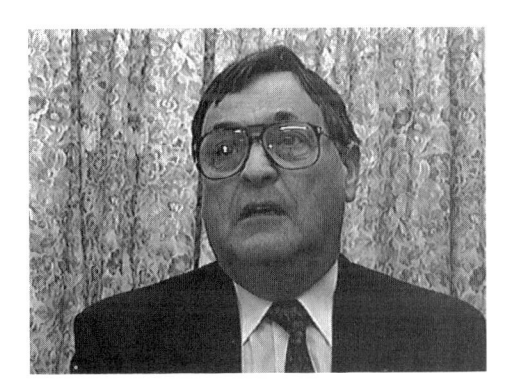

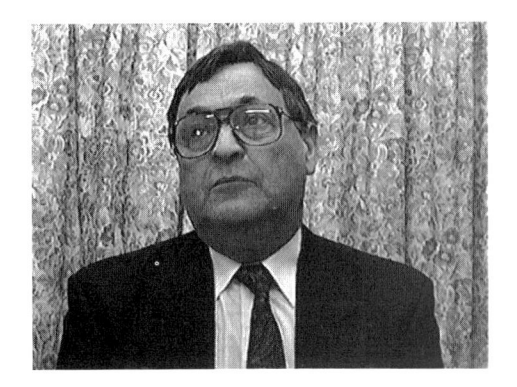

CSF fills the cerebral ventricles and subarachnoid spaces to form a buoyant, protective medium for the brain that reduces its 1.4-kg average mass to a weight of only 50 g. This allows the blood vessels, nerve roots and fine arachnoid trabeculae to anchor the brain effectively to the skull. CSF, which under normal circumstances has a composition similar to that of brain extracellular fluid, is made by the choroid plexus and also by cerebral vessels and the walls of the cerebral ventricles. Production within the ventricles, and absorption by the arachnoid villi into the cerebral venous sinuses at about $18\,mL\,h^{-1}$, leads to a flow of CSF out into the subarachnoid space through the midline foramen (of Magendie) and lateral foramina (of Luschka) of the fourth ventricle. The composition of CSF is similar in many ways to that of plasma, with the important exceptions that protein levels are normally very low (0.3% of plasma levels) and glucose is present at about 65% of blood levels. In addition, uric acid levels are one-third of plasma levels and lipids are virtually excluded.

Basic science

Blood–brain barrier

The observation that certain substances that pass freely from capillary blood into non-nervous tissues fail to pass from capillary blood into the tissues of the central nervous system led to the concept of the blood–brain barrier. The blood–brain barrier appears to be able to regulate the entry of macromolecular solutes, as well as lymphocytes and microbial pathogens, into the central nervous system. The identification of receptors within the brain substance for polar peptides such as growth hormone, that were originally thought to be excluded by the blood–brain barrier, has cast some doubt over the extent of the structure and placed further demands on the investigation of its selectivity and integrity under different disease states and in the presence of different pharmacological challenges. Similarly, as the central nervous system is not entirely isolated from the immune system by the blood–brain barrier, the brain is subject to modified immune surveillance. The exact nature and location of the blood–brain barrier—whether a special property of the endothelial cell layer of capillary walls or of the perivascular footplates of astrocytes on the basement membranes—remains a matter of conjecture, but the cells from which it is formed appear to contain continuous tight junctions and have very low rates of pinocytosis; hence its efficacy as an effective permeability barrier.

MCQs

1 CSF is generated by cerebral vessels and the walls of the cerebral ventricles.
2 The brain is anchored in the head by vascular pedicles, nerve roots and arachnoid trabeculae.
3 The composition of CSF is similar to that of plasma.
4 The blood–brain barrier excludes macromolecules from the central nervous system.
5 CSF is absorbed by the arachnoid villi at about $18\,mL\,h^{-1}$.

Case 27
Facial flushing and abdominal cramps

History

A 56-year-old businessman was seen in the outpatient department with a 10-month history of intermittent episodes of abdominal cramps and diarrhoea each lasting from 10 min to 6 h. The attacks had gradually increased in frequency and had occurred during the day and night. As some of the episodes seemed to be linked to eating, the diagnoses of irritable bowel syndrome and food allergy had both been suggested by his GP. The most recent episodes of abdominal pain had been accompanied by facial flushing. He denied any significant past medical history, but explained that, 15 years previously, a 25-cm length of small bowel had been resected for a 'benign' stricture.

On examination, his blood pressure was 136/84 mmHg. Auscultation of his chest revealed a pansystolic murmur. There were no neurological abnormalities or skin rash, the only findings of note being coarsening of the facial features, hepatomegaly (a smooth, non-tender liver edge extending 4 cm below the costal margin) and a paramedian laparotomy scar.

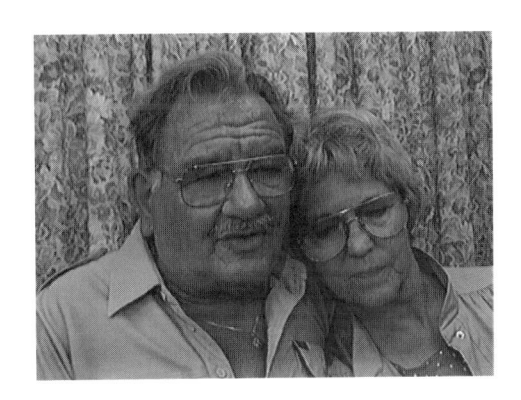

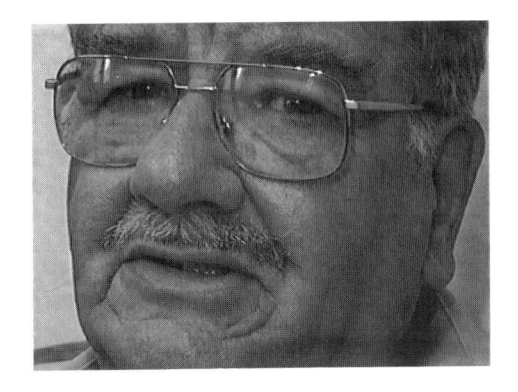

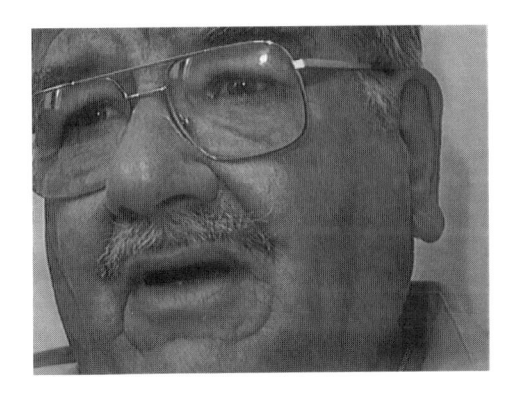

A full blood count, urea, electrolytes, plasma viscosity and liver function tests were within normal limits, except for a raised alkaline phosphatase level of 176 U L^{-1} (normal range = 20–120 U L^{-1}). His urinary 5-hydroxyindoleacetic acid (5-HIAA) level was 171.9 mmol per mole of creatinine (0–4 mmol per mole of creatinine). Hepatic ultrasound confirmed the presence of multiple cystic lesions, the largest being 7.2 cm in diameter. An echocardiogram showed tricuspid regurgitation. An electrocardiogram (ECG) was in sinus rhythm with a normal axis and no evidence of right atrial enlargement. An R wave in the right chest leads with T wave inversion suggested some right heart strain and right ventricular overload.

Notes

The patient had carcinoid syndrome.

When the previous records became available, the histology of the bowel resection 15 years previously was found to be 'carcinoid'. Carcinoid tumours, derived from enterochromaffin cells, are so-called because of their malignant-looking histology but relatively benign behaviour. They occur most commonly in the ileum, colon and structures derived from the embryonic foregut—the stomach, lungs, pancreas and thyroid. Paroxysmal secretion of 5-hydroxytryptamine (5-HT or serotonin) and other bioactive peptides by tumours draining into the hepatic portal system does not give rise to endocrine symptoms as the peptides are rapidly degraded by the liver (first pass metabolism). Once hepatic secondary deposits are present, however, direct drainage into the systemic circulation allows the peptides to exert their effects, producing characteristic episodes of abdominal cramp, diarrhoea and prolonged facial flushing, sometimes accompanied by tachycardia and, less commonly, by right-sided endocardial thickening with pulmonary valve stenosis or regurgitation. Patients with proven hepatic metastases from carcinoid tumours may live reasonably comfortably for many years. In this patient, an unsuccessful attempt was made to reduce the secretion or effects of 5-HT using somatostatin analogues and cyproheptadine, an antihistamine with pronounced anti-5-HT side-effects. Radiotherapy and chemotherapy are not useful in malignant carcinoid.

As metabolically active carcinoids cause malabsorption and anorexia, and tend to consume nicotinamide, vitamin supplements can be useful to prevent the development of pellagra.

Basic science

Pellagra

Nicotinic acid and nicotinamide are two forms of B vitamin (known as niacin in the USA) that form an essential part of nicotinamide adenine dinucleotide (NAD) and nicotinamide adenine dinucleotide phosphate (NADP), hydrogen-accepting coenzymes required for the utilization of food energy. In the oxidation–reduction reactions that characterize the metabolism of food, energy-rich electrons are stripped from food fuel (oxidation) and used to reduce adenosine diphosphate (ADP) to the more energy-rich adenosine triphosphate (ATP)—a universal, rapidly available energy source for other metabolic processes.

Oxidation–reduction reactions are cata-

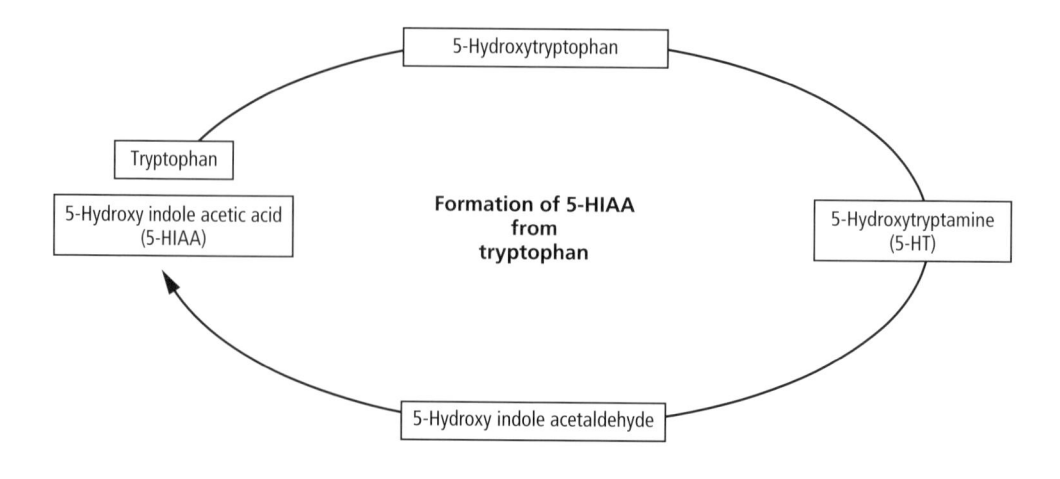

Formation of 5-HIAA from tryptophan

Tryptophan → 5-Hydroxytryptophan → 5-Hydroxytryptamine (5-HT) → 5-Hydroxy indole acetaldehyde → 5-Hydroxy indole acetic acid (5-HIAA)

lysed by two types of enzymes: 'oxidases' that transfer oxygen and 'dehydrogenases' that remove hydrogen atoms. Neither can hold on to the liberated hydrogen themselves and both therefore act with 'coenzymes' that can. NAD+ is an important coenzyme derived from nicotinic acid. Deficiency results in pellagra, characterized by a red, scaling photosensitive rash, patchy demyelination of the spinal cord and brain, and thickening of the gut and vaginal mucosa. The whole picture is characterized ultimately by the memorable triad of 'dermatitis, diarrhoea and dementia'.

Pellagra was once widespread in impoverished societies that subsisted entirely on maize, as the nicotinic acid that it contains remains bound and unavailable after normal cooking. Soaked in alkali, however (as it is during the production of Mexican tortillas), the vitamin is released, and being water soluble and heat resistant is readily absorbed and utilized. In Western society, pellagra is rare and tends to be confined to patients suffering from chronic malabsorption and alcoholics.

As tryptophan can be converted to nicotinic acid in the body (60 mg of the former produces 1 mg of the latter), foods containing tryptophan are included as 'nicotinic acid equivalents' in tables of food containing 'available' nicotinic acid. The recommended daily intake is 18 mg.

Table 27.1 Nicotinic acid content (mg per 100 g)

Instant coffee	45.7
Chicken	9.5
Beef	8.1
Fish	4.8
Bread	2.0
Milk	0.9

MCQs

1 Carcinoid syndrome is caused by excessive production of 5-HIAA.
2 Carcinoid syndrome is characterized by facial flushing, a right heart murmur and an abdominal mass.
3 Pellagra is characterized by dermatitis, diarrhoea and dementia.
4 Hepatic metastases in carcinoid syndrome indicate end-stage disease and death within 18 months.
5 Nicotinic acid is an essential component of NAD and NADP.

Case 28
Recurrent haematemesis

History

A 65-year-old housewife and former factory worker, with a past medical history of ischaemic heart disease and tuberculosis of the spine, was seen in hospital with a 4-year history of recurrent episodes of vomiting blood. In this respect, she had been well throughout her life until a sudden chest pain was followed by haematemesis. She described at least eight episodes of haematemesis, possibly associated with epistaxis, which eventually required 'endoscopy and laser treatment'. Gastro-oesophageal reflux had not been a problem and the patient had not suffered from 'indigestion' as far as she was aware. There was no family history of bleeding disorders.

On examination, she was noted to have Horner's syndrome and a sharply angled spinal kyphosis (gibbus) consistent with spinal tuberculosis. There were also a large number of telangiectases visible, particularly on her lips and hands.

Notes

The patient had hereditary haemorrhagic telangiectasia.

Hereditary haemorrhagic telangiectasia, or Osler–Rendu–Weber disease, is an inherited autosomal dominant condition in which frequent episodes of gastrointestinal and nasal bleeding occur from abnormal telangiectatic capillaries. Other conditions in which the integrity of vessel walls is compromised are scurvy (vitamin C deficiency), Cushing's syndrome (excessive glucocorticoid production), ageing (senile purpura), direct endothelial infection, such as the rickettsiae that cause Rocky Mountain spotted fever, disorders of connective tissue, such as Ehlers–Danlos syndrome, pseudoxanthoma elasticum and

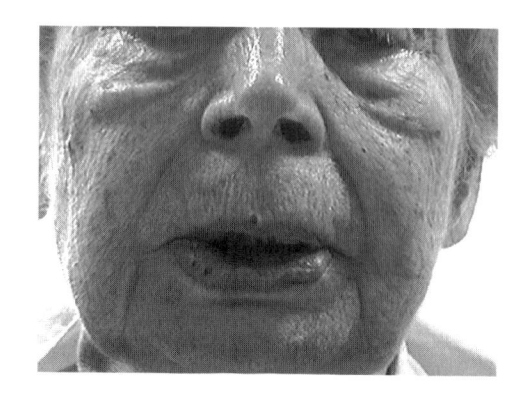

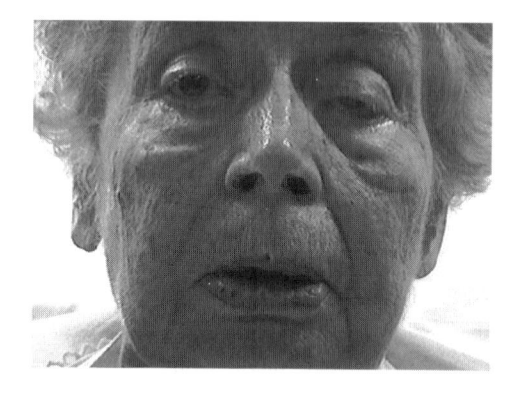

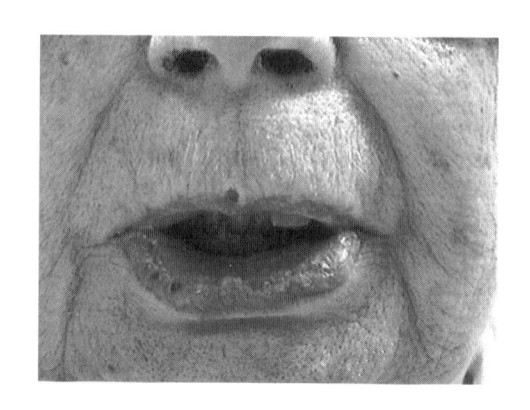

Marfan's syndrome, and other specific disorders, such as thrombotic thrombocytopenic purpura and Henoch–Schönlein purpura.

Basic science

Disorders of blood vessel walls

Vessel wall disorders are characterized by mild, but recurrent, bleeding from the skin and mucous membranes, typified by hereditary haemorrhagic telangiectasia. In many cases, classical tests of haemostasis are normal.

Thrombotic thrombocytopenic purpura. This is a fulminant disorder with a high mortality, possibly initiated by endothelial injury, that leads to the release of a series of coagulants and platelet aggregates from endothelial cells. The histological finding of microvascular deposition of thrombi without surrounding inflammation is diagnostic (often identified in gingival biopsies) and is usually accompanied by thrombocytopenia, fever, renal failure, microangiopathic haemolytic anaemia and fluctuating levels of consciousness with variable neurological signs. Disseminated intravascular coagulation is not a feature of this condition.

Haemolytic uraemic syndrome. A disease of early childhood, characterized by fever, thrombocytopenia, microangiopathic haemolytic anaemia, hypertension and acute renal failure, that resembles thrombotic thrombocytopenic purpura. Unlike thrombotic thrombocytopenic purpura, however, the disease is limited to the kidneys.

Henoch–Schönlein purpura. This is a distinctive, self-limiting vasculitis which occurs in children and young adults, often preceded by upper respiratory tract infection of streptococcal pharyngitis. It is characterized by an acute inflammatory reaction with immunoglobulin A (IgA) and complement deposition in capillaries, small arterioles and renal mesangial tissues. The inflammation increases vascular permeability and leads to haemorrhage and exudates. A purpuric or urticarial rash occurs on the extensor surfaces of the arms and legs, and particularly on the buttocks, associated with colicky abdominal pain, haematuria from glomerulonephritis and arthralgia or polyarthritis.

MCQs

1. Hereditary haemorrhagic telangiectasia is inherited as an autosomal dominant condition.
2. Recurrent, severe bleeding into muscles and joints is typical of vessel wall disorders.
3. Henoch–Schönlein purpura is often preceded by a streptococcal upper respiratory tract infection.
4. Thrombotic thrombocytopenic purpura is characterized by severe disseminated intravascular coagulation.
5. The telangiectases in hereditary haemorrhagic telangiectasia are confined to mucous membranes.

Case 29
Weight loss and itching

History

A 77-year-old former catering assistant was admitted to hospital with a 2-year history of lethargy and weight loss. Close questioning revealed that her 'taste for food' had declined and that, when she did eat, she felt full after ingesting a relatively small amount. Several months after the start of the weight loss, she had begun to itch all over her scalp and back, and had frequently excoriated her skin with her fingernails in an attempt to ameliorate it without much success. Her only other symptom was chronic back pain associated with some loss of height and the development of a mild kyphosis. She denied any changes in the colour of her urine or stools, or a history of jaundice at any time.

On examination, she was anxious and tired, clinically anaemic and had clearly lost a considerable amount of weight. Her skin showed scratch marks in keeping with her history, and her liver was firm and smoothly enlarged. Investigations revealed an increased immunoglobulin M (IgM) level and positive anti-mitochondrial antibodies, together with a markedly elevated alkaline phosphatase level and modestly elevated transaminases. Her calcium level was 2.1 mmol L^{-1} (normal range = 2.12–2.62 mmol L^{-1}) with a low to normal phosphate level.

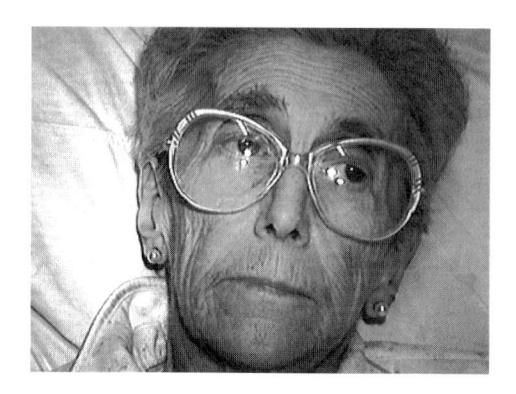

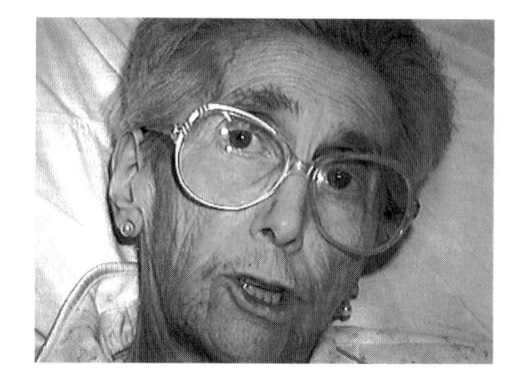

Notes

The patient had primary biliary cirrhosis.

The underlying cause of primary biliary cirrhosis remains unknown. There is a strong predilection for the condition to affect middle-aged women (90%) and, as the disease is loosely associated with other autoimmune conditions, 95% of cases are associated with the presence of an IgG antimitochondrial antibody and at least 80% of cases are associated with elevated serum IgM levels, an autoimmune aetiology seems likely.

Primary biliary cirrhosis is a diffuse, non-suppurative cholangitis that progressively destroys medium and small bile ducts over a period of months to several years. The process leads to cirrhosis, loss of hepatocytes and increasing biliary stasis. The first clinical signs are usually persistent, generalized itching, followed by the development of dark urine, pale stools and jaundice. Absence of bile leads to fat and fat-soluble vitamin malabsorption, with steatorrhoea, purpura (vitamin K malabsorption prolonging clotting time) and osteomalacia (vitamin D malabsorption), leading to backache and bone pain.

Fatigue is a non-specific, but disabling, symptom that affects up to two-thirds of patients with primary biliary cirrhosis. Pruritus is another common and often distressing symptom of liver and biliary tract disorders. Its pathogenesis is unknown, although a variety of drugs that reduce the concentration of a number of substances (including, presumably, one or more undefined pruritogens—perhaps bile acids and bile salts), such as cholestyramine and colestipol, can partially ameliorate the symptom. Recent evidence suggests that the perception of itching is mediated by endogenous opioids, an observation that explains the success of opiate antagonists as adjunctive therapy in alleviating the condition.

Basic science

Bile and gallstones

Hepatic bile is a pigmented, isotonic fluid, similar to plasma in electrolyte composition, and secreted into the biliary tree at a rate of around 500 mL per 24 h by a secretin-responsive, cyclic adenosine monophosphate (cAMP)-dependent mechanism. Once in the gall-bladder, much of the salts are reabsorbed, leaving an aqueous solution containing 12% bile acids (cholic and chenodeoxycholic acids, synthesized from cholesterol, which have powerful detergent activity and form molecular aggregates called micelles), 4% phospholipids and 0.7% unesterified cholesterol (kept in suspension by bile acids), as well as very small amounts of conjugated bilirubin, mucus, proteins and drugs. Conjugated and unconjugated bile acids are reabsorbed passively by the gut, and are taken up from the bloodstream by hepatocytes, which reconjugate them and secrete them once again into the bile. In this way, the whole bile acid pool (of about 4 g) is circulated several times a day, with losses of about 0.5 g daily into the stool, compensated for by *de novo* synthesis.

In the fasting state, the sphincter of Oddi closes the common bile duct and promotes filling of the gall-bladder with bile. Cholecystokinin, released from the duodenal mucosa in response to the ingestion of fats and amino acids, causes gall-bladder contraction, relaxation of the sphincter of Oddi and flow of bile into the duodenum. Gallstones develop in one in three women and one in five men, and at least two-thirds remain asymptomatic. Cholesterol is the chief component in 75%, the remaining 25% consisting mostly of bile pigments with or without calcium salts. Most gallstones originate in the gall-bladder, and symptoms are absent or only occur after a fatty meal. If stones originate in the common bile duct or pass into there from the gall-bladder, the symptoms are more severe and the risk of major illness is much higher.

Gall-bladder pain is usually a severe pain localized to the right upper quadrant or the upper part of the abdomen, lasting for at least 30 min. In cholecystitis, the pain is severe and accompanied by fever, nausea, vomiting and, if the cause is stones in the common bile duct, jaundice. An ultrasound of the gall-bladder and biliary tree will usually show dilatation of the common duct, and endoscopic retrograde cholangiography can be used to confirm the finding.

Drugs such as long-acting somatostatin analogues, used to treat carcinoid syndrome or acromegaly, markedly predispose to gallstone formation, as does obesity and gastric bypass surgery to treat it. Oral bile acids in the form of ursodeoxycholic acid or chenodeoxycholic acid can be given to dissolve radiolucent cholesterol stones, but act very slowly, obviating their use in severe disease.

MCQs

1 Primary biliary cirrhosis produces focal cholangitis leading to cirrhosis.
2 Itching is often one of the most prominent

and earliest symptoms of primary biliary cirrhosis.
3 Much of the cholesterol content of bile is reabsorbed by the gallbladder.
4 Bile salts undergo enterohepatic recirculation a number of times each day.
5 Most patients with gallstones eventually become symptomatic.

Case 30
Jaundice and poor coordination

History

A 21-year-old man was seen in hospital for stabilization of worsening ataxia and dysarthria. The problem first became manifest at the age of 12 years, when he developed clumsiness and was noted by his GP to be mildly jaundiced. He was referred to hospital where, in addition to jaundice, he was found to have choreoathetoid movements of his limbs. Further history excluded exposure to known cases of hepatitis or foreign travel, and he had not been taking any drugs at the time. Ophthalmic examination at the bedside, including fundoscopy, was normal. A liver biopsy showed cirrhosis without evidence of hepatitis. Hepatitis serology was negative and α_1-antitrypsin levels were normal, but his bilirubin level was elevated at 65 µmol L^{-1} (normal range <17 µmol L^{-1}) with an aspartate aminotransferase level of 77 U L^{-1} (6–35 U L^{-1}) and alkaline phosphatase level of 119 U L^{-1} (20–120 U L^{-1}). His sister was found to have the same condition, but to have few clinical effects. Treatment with penicillamine produced a marked improvement in his symptoms initially, and he began to train in banking and commerce. He failed to comply with treatment during the turbulent and rebellious years of his adolescence, unfortunately, and his symptoms worsened once again.

Notes

The patient had Wilson's disease.

Careful slit lamp examination revealed Kayser–Fleischer rings, and a ceruloplasmin level was reported as less than 0.07 g L^{-1} (0.15–0.6 g L^{-1}) with a serum copper level of 2.9 µmol L^{-1} (13–24 µmol L^{-1}).

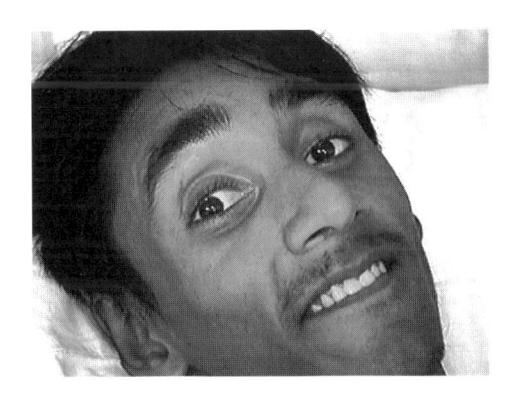

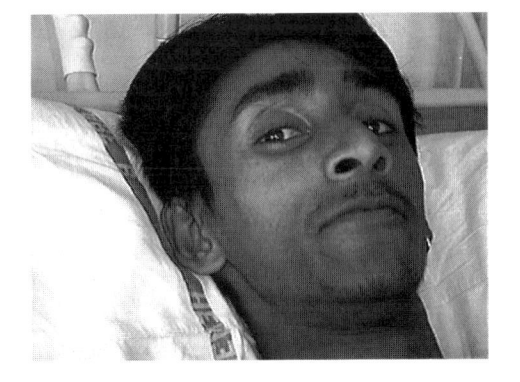

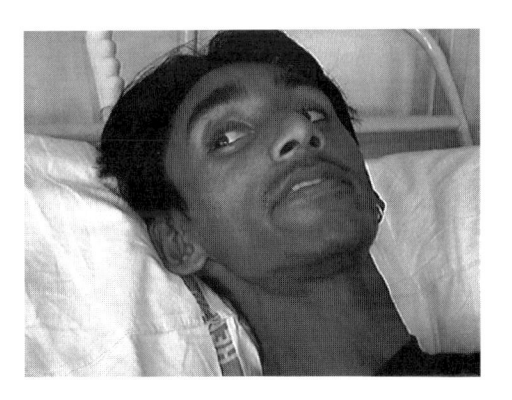

Wilson's disease is an autosomal recessive condition resulting from inactivating mutations of a copper-transporting P-type ATPase (ATP7B) on chromosome 13. The result of the condition, which has a prevalence of about 30 per million worldwide, is the accumulation of copper in the liver and, subsequently, in the brain and other organs. The more disrupted the function of the gene, the more severe the phenotype. The characteristic biochemical feature is a low level of the copper-carrying plasma protein ceruloplasmin. Persistent high levels of hepatic copper usually produce symptoms in childhood (from the age of 6 years until late adolescence) that may mimic other conditions, such as infectious mononucleosis, chronic active hepatitis and cirrhosis, or produce fulminant hepatic failure. The first signs of liver involvement may be the development of cirrhosis.

Psychiatric symptoms (perhaps contributing to his failure to comply with treatment) and neurological signs, such as tremor, spasticity, dysarthria, dysphagia and chorea, are commonly associated with Wilson's disease.

Basic science

Copper metabolism

Copper is a normal component of a number of enzymes, such as cytochrome oxidase, superoxide dismutase and tyrosinase. It is required for the synthesis of haemoglobin and is an essential component of myelin. Dietary sources of copper include shellfish, legumes, meat, liver and whole grains, and the normal daily intake is around 3.5 mg, with a total body content of around 70 mg. Copper deficiency is rare and almost confined to infants fed for prolonged periods with cows' milk only.

Under normal conditions, copper accumulation is prevented by the catabolic cleavage of copper from its carrier protein ceruloplasmin in the liver, and excretion into the bile. In Wilson's disease, hepatic lysosomes appear to be unable to excrete the free copper into the bile. Excess copper prevents the formation of ceruloplasmin from apoceruloplasmin and copper, and, once hepatocyte copper storage capacity is exceeded, it is released into the blood and taken up by other tissues, such as the kidneys, where it does not appear to cause toxic effects, and the brain, where it does. If tolerated, long-term treatment with penicillamine can prevent the manifestations of the disease.

MCQs

1 In Wilson's disease, serum copper levels are raised.
2 Kayser–Fleischer rings are always present in Wilson's disease patients with neurological damage.
3 The symptoms and signs of Wilson's disease are usually manifest before the age of 6 years.
4 In Wilson's disease, serum ceruloplasmin levels are usually low.
5 A course of penicillamine to remove excess copper gives lifelong protection.

Case 31
The woman who giggled on the phone

History

A 46-year-old woman was admitted, as far as she was concerned, fit and well. For some months, her employer, for whom she worked as a credit control manager, had been concerned about her performance and health. Her family too had been concerned, but had not acted until the patient had an episode of uncontrolled giggling during a telephone call. Her sister asked her to call her back, and when she did, once again, all the patient was able to do was giggle incoherently. This behaviour was so uncharacteristic that her family rushed her to her doctor and she was admitted for further investigations. Still having very little insight into her problem, the patient nevertheless realized that something must be wrong to have caused the giggling and complied with the advice of her family and medical attendants.

There were no abnormal findings on examination. In particular, there were no skin stigmata of neurofibromatosis, no hepatomegaly and no splenomegaly or lymphadenopathy. Breast examination was normal. No abnormal signs were detected on examination of her central or peripheral nervous system. A CT scan of her head was carried out.

Notes

The patient had a large frontal lobe meningioma.

Tumours of the frontal lobes can attain a considerable size before unequivocal signs of cerebral impairment develop. Even then, they can be very subtle, with progressive disturbance of thought processes, reduced insight and loss of business acumen, poor memory and lethargy. Urinary incontinence and disordered gait may also become evident.

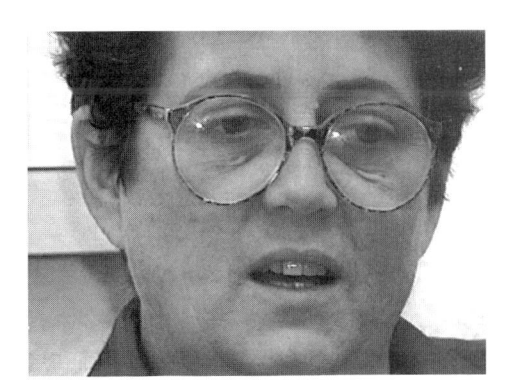

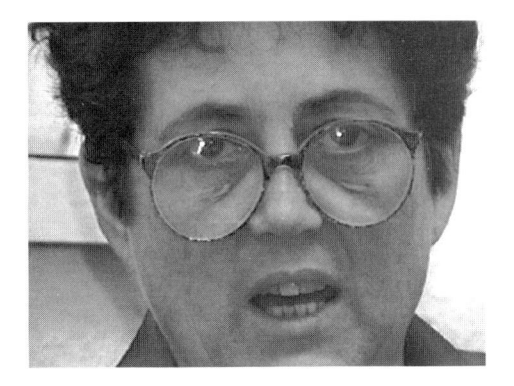

Basic science

Brain tumours

Primary brain tumours arise from glial cells (astrocytomas (10% of total), oligodendrogliomas (1% of total) and glioblastomas (20% of total)), supporting tissues (meningiomas (20% of total) or schwannomas) or ependymal cells (ependymomas). In children, more primitive tumours, such as neuroblastomas, medulloblastomas and chordomas, are also prevalent. Metastases from extracranial neoplasms account for 23% of intracranial tumours.

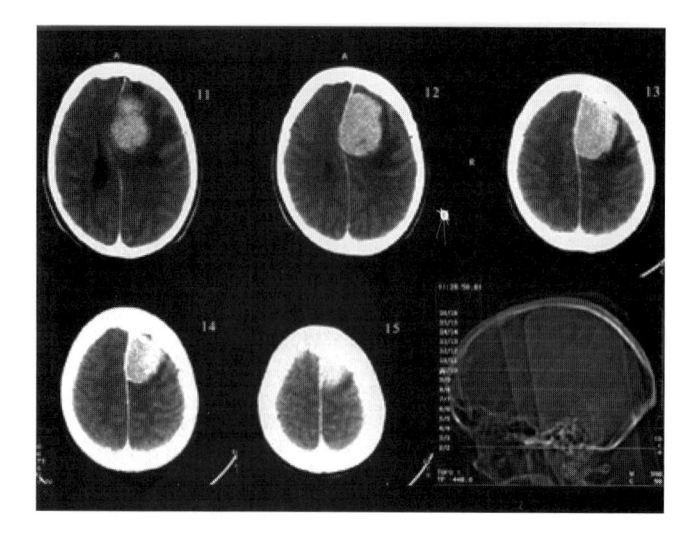

Intracranial tumours can be either within the brain tissue or compress the brain from outside. Slow growth can be accommodated by the brain, but masses more than 3 cm in diameter tend to compress the brain and compromise its blood supply and cerebrospinal fluid (CSF) pathways—exacerbated by concurrent oedema.

Headache and vomiting with minimal nausea are characteristic signs that occur in ≤50% of patients, and a decline in cognitive or neurological function can occur, together with the onset of epilepsy, which is the first sign in 20% of intracranial neoplasms.

MCQs

1 Epilepsy is the first sign in 20% of intracranial neoplasms.
2 Metastases from extracranial neoplasms account for the majority of brain tumours.
3 Frontal lobe tumours tend to present early, usually before they are 1 cm in diameter.
4 Meningiomas account for 50% of intracranial neoplasms.
5 Slow growing intracranial masses frequently reach 10 cm in diameter before the onset of symptoms.

Case 32
Slurred speech and choking

History

A 54-year-old unemployed gardener and former dock worker was admitted to hospital at the request of his sister and the staff of his warden-assisted residence with an 18-month history of weight loss and difficulty in swallowing. The patient himself was unable to provide a history and, although alert and apparently orientated, could not speak — a problem that was initially considered to be a manifestation of depression. His sister provided a history for him that started with headaches and a persistent cough, followed by the gradual onset of dysphagia and slurred speech. Despite frequent attendances at the GP's surgery, a referral for an ear, nose and throat (ENT) opinion and the suggestion by his sister (a nurse) that the problem seemed to be neurological, no diagnosis was made. The dysphagia gradually worsened, and his speech became so indistinct that he was unable to communicate except in grunts. At the same time, his family noted that he was becoming physically weak and that, when dropped at the end of his road rather than right at his front door, he became distressed. As the dysphagia worsened, he rapidly lost weight and was eventually referred to hospital where a diagnosis was made in casualty.

On examination, the most significant findings were confined to the nervous system. He was noted to have mild, asymmetrical weakness of his arms and legs and to take a considerable time to assume a sitting posture from lying. Tendon reflexes were brisk, and widespread fasciculation was noted on examination of his limb muscles. His tongue was spastic and fasciculating; swallowing was severely impaired. No sensory changes were detectable, although examination was difficult.

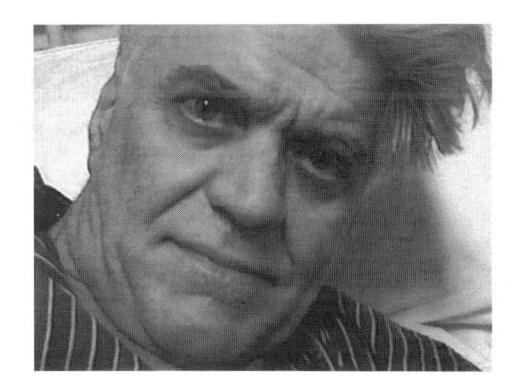

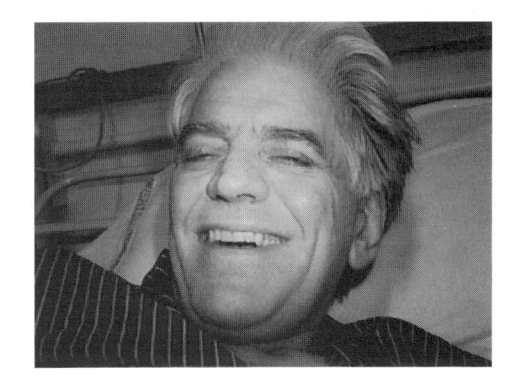

The diagnosis was confirmed electromyographically.

Notes

The patient had motor neurone disease.

Needle electromyographs recorded from the right tibialis anterior and the vastus lateralis showed frequent fibrillation, sharp waves and fasciculations, together with an excess of polyphasic units and reduced interference patterns consistent with motor neurone disease. The examination was brief because the patient had trouble tolerating the investigation.

Amyotrophic lateral sclerosis is the most frequent presentation of motor neurone disease. The condition usually affects patients in late middle age and affects men more often than women. In fewer than 10% of cases, the condition is transmitted in an autosomal dominant fashion. The characteristic feature of the condition is progressive non-inflammatory degenerative loss of the upper motor neurones of the cerebral cortex and brain stem, and the lower motor neurone anterior horn cells. Initially, the disease may be confined to the anterior horn cells, leading to progressive muscular denervation and muscle cell atrophy (hence 'amyotrophy'), or to the brain stem, leading to progressive bulbar palsy. Involvement of the upper motor neurones of the cortex leads to their replacement in the internal capsule and pyramids of the medulla with glial tissue. This imparts a firmness to the corticospinal tracts in the brain stem (hence 'lateral sclerosis'). The result is pseudobulbar palsy and increased tendon reflexes as seen in the present patient. In addition to the muscles of the face and tongue and the muscles used for chewing and swallowing, the respiratory muscles are affected and may lead to death. Curiously, intellect, the sensory nervous system and the nerves responsible for urinary and faecal continence, the nerve supply to the extraocular muscles and the mechanisms that control and coordinate movement remain entirely intact.

Basic science

Motor function

Motor function is subserved by the primary motor area—the cerebral cortex that lies immediately in front of the precentral sulcus, the structure that separates the frontal lobe from the parietal lobe. It receives inputs from the premotor cortex anteriorly, the thalamus inferiorly and the sensory cortex posteriorly. Innervation from the motor cortex is contralateral to the limbs, but has a significant ipsilateral and bilateral input to the head, neck and axial musculature.

Fibres from the motor cortex begin to come together in the corona radiata, form a compact band in the internal capsule and descend into the brain stem. As the tracts continue down through the ventral medulla, they form the pyramids (hence the synonym 'pyramidal' tract). Most of the fibres cross over at the decussation of the pyramids and continue their descent as the lateral corticospinal tract, synapsing on lower motor neurones in the anterior horn. The fibres that synapse in the motor nuclei of the brain stem are so-called 'corticobulbar fibres'. Those that continue ipsilaterally into the spinal cord, become the ventral corticospinal tract.

MCQs

1 Degenerative changes in motor neurone disease are limited to upper motor neurones.
2 Amyotrophic lateral sclerosis is usually transmitted in an autosomal dominant fashion.
3 In motor neurone disease, involvement of nerves to the extraocular muscles leads to diplopia.
4 Urinary and faecal incontinence can complicate terminal motor neurone disease.
5 The primary motor cortex is located in the parietal lobe.

Case 33
An accident on the way to the airport

History

A 28-year-old sales manager in a boutique presented to her doctor with a history of severe upper backache, without exacerbating or relieving factors, that had come on quite suddenly and waxed and waned in severity over 6 months. Examination of her back on a number of occasions was unremarkable, and she was reassured by her GP that the most likely cause of her symptoms was a pulled muscle. The pain at the top of her back abated with time, but she subsequently suffered lower back pain and bouts of abdominal pains and nausea that her doctor was unable to explain. Some months later, the patient suffered an episode of transient loss of bowel control. She was on her way to the airport for a holiday in Portugal with her husband and, as she felt otherwise well, put the episode down to being 'overexcited and stressed'. Much to her alarm and embarrassment, a similar accident occurred while she was on holiday. After returning to the UK, she began to notice that she had become slightly more clumsy, and that, when trying to walk between two customers in the shop, she invariably bumped into one or the other. Otherwise she claimed to be perfectly well, although increasingly concerned about her symptoms and fearful of humiliating herself. Because of the latter, she persuaded her doctor to refer her to a specialist, and was seen in neurology outpatients where a neurological examination revealed marked loss of pain sensation in her legs extending onto her trunk. Cranial nerve examination was normal. A magnetic resonance imaging (MRI) scan of the spinal cord revealed the diagnosis.

Notes

A series of syrinxes was seen on MRI scan. At

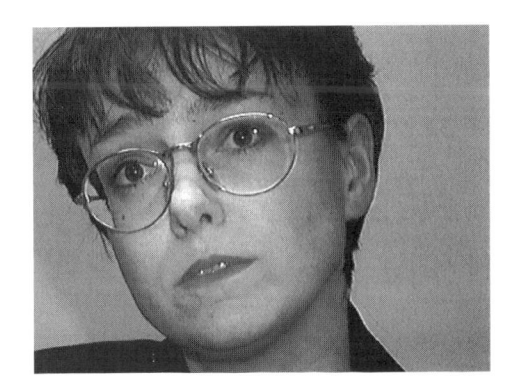

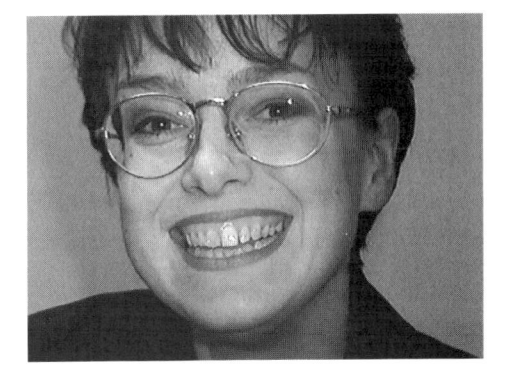

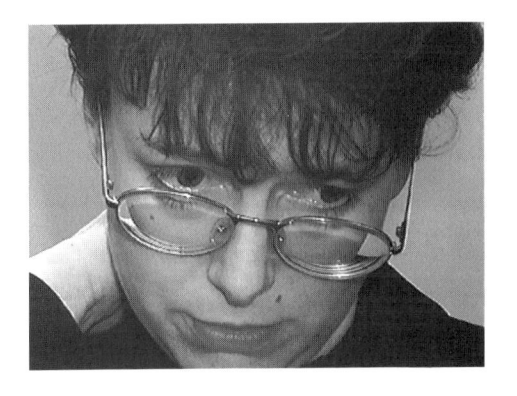

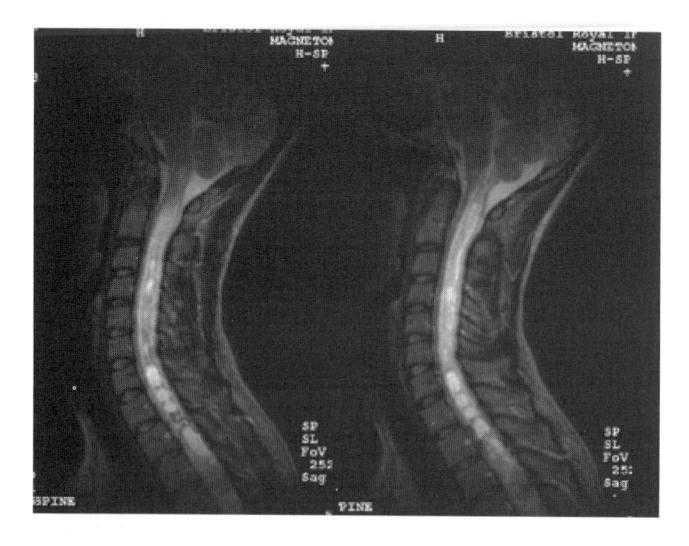

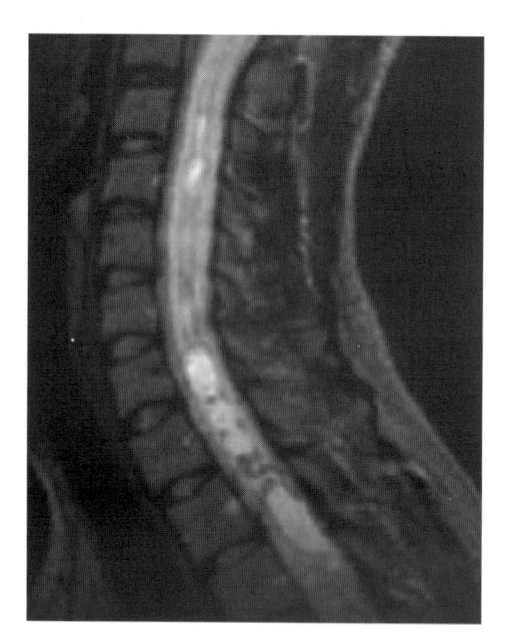

neurosurgery, the cause of syringomyelia was found to be a haemangioblastoma obstructing cerebrospinal fluid (CSF) flow, which was successfully resected.

Ballooning of the central cavity of the spinal cord is, in most cases, associated with a mild degree of Arnold–Chiari malformation in which the cerebellar tonsils lie in the posterior aspect of the foramen magnum and transmit increased CSF pressure (for example, when straining, coughing or sneezing) into the central canal instead of the spinal CSF. The development of slit-like dissections adjacent to the enlargement of the central canal can be responsible for the asymmetry of signs, and the acute development or worsening of signs can occur in some patients following a cough or sneeze. The expansion usually begins at C7–T1, and from this level can spread up to the face to give sensory loss in the distribution of a Balaclava helmet.

Not infrequently, the syndrome occurs secondary to an obstructing tumour, and, in this case, a haemangioblastoma was found and the diagnosis of von Hippel–Lindau syndrome was contemplated.

Basic science

Neural control of bladder and bowels

Micturition. The neural control of micturition is not very well understood. The bladder contains stretch receptors that, when activated, form the afferent limb of a reflex arc based on the S3 nerve roots and S3 segment of the cord. The efferent loop is mediated by parasympathetic efferents to the smooth muscle of the bladder wall. A sympathetic nerve supply from the hypogastric plexus runs to the urethral sphincter mechanism. This reflex arc results in intermittent, involuntary micturition in unconscious patients, in infancy and after various lesions of the nervous system, such as spinal cord compression. Voluntary inhibition of micturition involves inhibition of the reflex arc described above mediated by an area in the frontal lobe through motor fibres in or adjacent to the corticospinal tract. Micturition itself involves complete volitional relaxation of the external sphincter and relaxation of the pelvic floor so that reflex detrusor contraction (which pulls open the bladder neck) can occur. This is often accompanied by a reflex Valsalva's manoeuvre to increase intra-abdominal pressure and hasten micturition.

A frontal lobe lesion may cause sudden, uncontrolled micturition with no residual volume (and no concern, depending on accompanying problems). Spinal cord damage leads to a small, spastic bladder, sudden, but often incomplete bladder emptying and lack of appreciation of bladder fullness. Disruption of the sacral reflex loop by cauda equina damage or damage to the nerves in the pelvis leads to continuous, dribbling incontinence with no sensation of bladder fullness and poor emptying. Loss of perineal sensation and sexual function also occur. Loss of nerve function within the bladder wall (found, for example, in subacute combined degeneration, diabetes mellitus and multiple sclerosis) causes massive urinary retention and dribbling incontinence with a high risk of infection.

Defaecation. Mass movement of faeces within the colon causes acute distension of the rectum and initiates the defaecatory reflex. Defaecation is consciously prevented by voluntary contraction of the striated muscle of the pelvic floor and the external anal sphincter. If allowed to proceed, contractions of the rectum and sigmoid increase pressure in the rectum and also reduce the rectosigmoidal angle. Relaxation of the internal and external anal sphincters then permits the evacuation of faeces. Spinal cord damage reduces the sensation of rectal distension and reduces anal tone, allowing the involuntary evacuation of faeces, particularly if intra-abdominal pressure is raised.

MCQs

1 The Arnold–Chiari malformation predisposes to syringomyelia.
2 The neurological deficits produced by syringomyelia can worsen in seconds.
3 Detrusor muscle contraction during micturition is mediated by sympathetic inputs.
4 Intermittent involuntary micturition can occur after spinal cord section.
5 Micturition involves contraction of the pelvic floor.

Case 34
Eye make up!

History

A 42-year-old woman was seen in the outpatient department with tingling and numbness of the left side of her face that had come on overnight. The previous day she had applied some eye make up and, to her surprise, found that she had accidentally put some eyelash thickener onto her cornea. The following morning she woke up to find that her upper lip was 'tingling' and that the whole left side of her face was numb. She denied biting her tongue and claimed that the sensation in her mouth was entirely normal. Her past medical history was of transphenoidal surgery for a pituitary adenoma 17 years previously, followed by pituitary radiotherapy. She was otherwise well.

On examination of her cranial nerves, the only abnormal finding was that all modalities of facial sensation were absent on the left hand side almost to the midline, extending to the vertex and chin, excluding an area of the angle of the mandible. Her corneal reflex was absent on the left. Hearing was normal bilaterally, as were her visual fields to confrontation.

Notes

The patient had developed a left-sided trigeminal nerve palsy. No reason was found and, in the absence of other diagnoses, the changes were attributed to collateral damage from pituitary radiotherapy, an exceedingly rare complication.

Direct damage to the trigeminal nerve is unusual. When it occurs, it is usually the result of one of the following conditions:
- Herpes zoster (which has a particular predilection to the ophthalmic division).
- Multiple sclerosis.
- Trigeminal neuralgia (in which the attack of

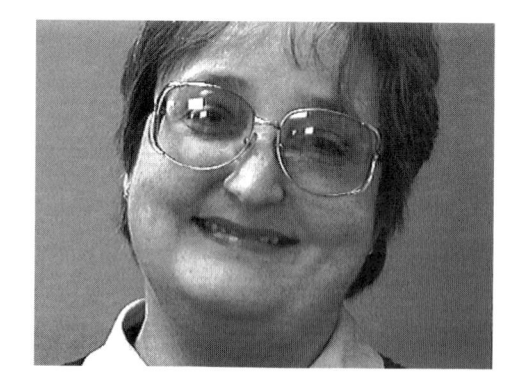

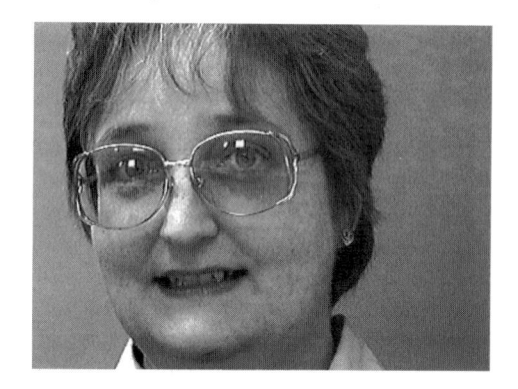

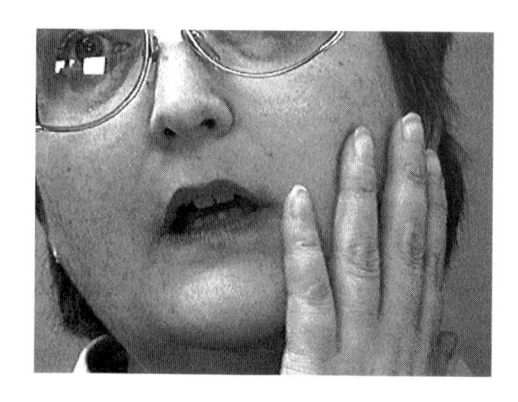

pain is sometimes followed by transient numbness).
- Trigeminal sensory neuropathy (in which the numbness is progressive).
- Tumours of the nasopharynx.
- Displacement of the trigeminal ganglion:
    Acoustic neuroma.
    Aneurysm of the basilar artery.
    Meningioma or other tumour.

The clinical effects may initially be very subtle, with abolition of the corneal reflex only. Loss of facial sensation may eventually follow.

Basic science

Trigeminal nerve

The trigeminal nerve is the principal sensory nerve for the head and the motor nerve for muscles of mastication. The extent of sensory innervation is highly significant clinically, as facial numbness is a common symptom in patients with functional rather than organic disease. The important features are as follows.

- The ophthalmic division of the trigeminal nerve extends to the vertex (uppermost part of the head) or just beyond, rather than, as many patients believe, the hairline.
- As all axial sensory nerves interdigitate in the midline, in unilateral sensory nerve palsy, the line of sensory loss should be a few millimetres from the midline, towards the affected side.
- The corneal reflex, tested by touching the cornea (not the sclera or eyelashes) to one side of the pupil (so that the sight of an object does not induce a blink) with a wisp of cotton wool, is difficult to resist and is an excellent sign of intact innervation.
- The region of skin over the angle of the jaw is innervated by branches from C2 and C3, not the mandibular division of the trigeminal nerve. Thus, in trigeminal palsy, the sensation over this area should be preserved.
- The motor component of the trigeminal nerve, in addition to the muscles of mastication, includes the tensor tympani, tensor veli palatini, anterior belly of digastric and mylohyoid muscles. The significant bilateral innervation to the motor nuclei of the trigeminal nerve tends to make the assessment of motor function less informative than that of sensory function.

MCQs

1 Facial nerve palsy is part of the differential diagnosis of objective facial sensory loss.
2 The facial sensory loss in trigeminal nerve palsy extends to the hairline.
3 The myelin of myelinated nerves is contained within Schwann cell membranes.
4 Loss of corneal sensation is characteristic of facial nerve damage.
5 Sensory loss over the angle of the jaw is found in trigeminal palsy.

Case 35
The foot that flapped

History

A 59-year-old housewife with insulin-dependent diabetes mellitus was seen in clinic with a 3-day history of pain and weakness in the right leg. Having previously been completely well, she noticed that her right foot appeared to be 'flapping', and that she was automatically lifting her right leg higher than normal to avoid tripping over while walking to the newsagents. Thinking that her flat shoes were responsible, she returned home and changed to higher heels, but this did not seem to help. Several hours later, she developed numbness and then pain on the outside of her right calf, extending down over the dorsum and underside of her right foot. She had a past history of insulin-dependent diabetes mellitus diagnosed 30 years previously and, 20 years before her current presentation, an episode of severe back pain extending down both thighs attributed to sciatica. This took 5.5 months to resolve, and was not associated at the time or subsequently with muscle weakness, numbness or paraesthesia.

Notes

The patient had diabetic mononeuropathy affecting the common peroneal nerve.

Investigations which included lumbar puncture and spinal magnetic resonance imaging did not reveal any other specific pathology. The cause of neuropathy in diabetes is still unclear. Current evidence suggests that sorbitol, the product of glucose metabolism by the enzyme aldose reductase, displaces taurine, an osmolyte and antioxidant, from nerve cells and renders them more susceptible to damage. New, powerful aldose reductase inhibitors may afford some protection against diabetic neuropathy in the future.

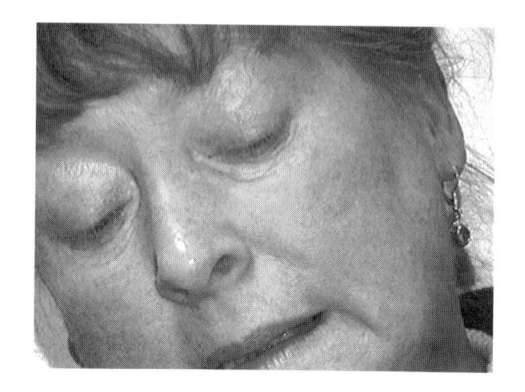

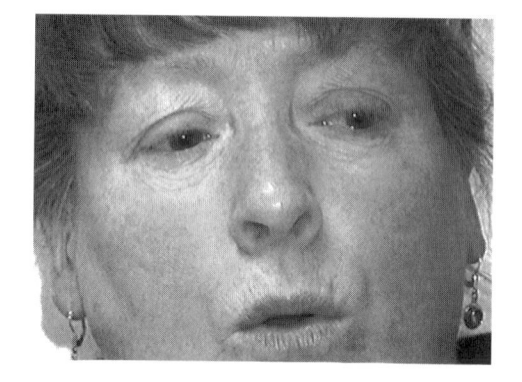

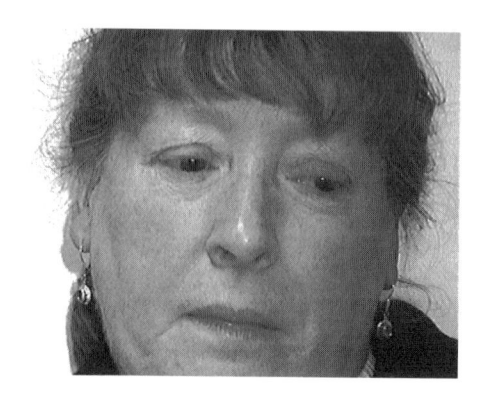

The common peroneal nerve is one of the terminal divisions of the sciatic nerve in the popliteal fossa. It supplies the muscles that dorsiflex the toes and dorsiflex and evert the foot, as well as sensation to the dorsum of the foot and lateral aspect of the lower half of the leg. Pressure damage, particularly of the part overlying the head of the fibula, is the most frequent type of injury, but it is also involved in fractures of the upper part of the fibula, diabetic neuropathy, polyarteritis nodosa and knee surgery. Foot drop may be an early sign in certain types of muscular dystrophy, such as facioscapulohumeral muscular dystrophy, caused by weakness of the peroneal and anterior tibial muscles.

Basic science

Mononeuropathy is injury to a single nerve trunk. Direct trauma is usually self-evident, but the effects of compression, which is often the mechanism responsible, can be more insidious and difficult to detect. Mononeuropathy involving the median nerve, for example, can occur in association with a Colles' fracture at the wrist or in the axilla from dislocation of the shoulder, but is usually the result of chronic compression in the carpal tunnel.

Mononeuritis multiplex is the simultaneous or sequential involvement of a number of nerve trunks over days or years. The initial pattern of involvement is characteristically patchy but, as further nerves become involved, the distribution often becomes more symmetrical. In most cases, axonal degeneration is thought to be responsible, but demyelination as part of a chronic, acquired demyelinating neuropathy is involved in one-third of cases. In clinical practice, the most common underlying cause is diabetes mellitus. Sarcoidosis, amyloidosis and causes of nerve ischaemia, such as cryoglobulinaemia, Sjögren's syndrome, Wegener's granulomatosis and systemic sclerosis, are also sometimes implicated.

Involvement of the musculocutaneous nerve denervates the biceps and brachialis muscle and results in weak elbow flexion. Involvement of the lateral femoral cutaneous nerve results in pain involving the lateral aspect of the thigh (meralgia paraesthetica), and the ulnar nerve is particularly susceptible to compression in the ulnar groove on the extensor surface of the elbow. Isolated lesions of the radial nerve, suprascapular nerve, long thoracic nerve, brachial or lumbosacral plexus, obturator, femoral, tibial or sciatic nerves are also well described. Bell's palsy is the result of idiopathic facial nerve inflammation in the facial canal, and herpes zoster causes a sensory neuritis of one or more dorsal root ganglia.

MCQs

1 The common peroneal nerve is one of the terminal branches of the femoral nerve.
2 The common peroneal nerve is most commonly damaged by direct pressure.
3 The most common cause of mononeuritis multiplex is diabetes mellitus.
4 Foot drop may be an early sign of muscular dystrophy.
5 Meralgia paraesthetica produces pain over the lateral aspect of the thigh.

Case 36
Dizziness and haematemesis

History

A 63-year-old housewife and mother was seen in accident and emergency with a short history of dizziness and vomiting blood. She had been completely well until the day of admission, had retired to bed as usual, woken at her normal time the following morning and was listening to the radio in bed before getting up. Several minutes later, she suddenly felt 'dizzy', became markedly nauseated and vomited copiously several times. Towards the end of the vomiting, she noticed a small amount of fresh red blood. After about 20 min, the acute vertigo and nausea waned. The patient denied drinking alcohol or smoking, and had not experienced any tinnitus or acute deafness. She had no previous history of similar episodes and no history of migraine or significant past medical events.

The abnormal findings on examination were marked obesity (present since childhood) and nystagmus to the right, which gradually resolved within 90 min of admission. Cranial nerve examination, including Rinne's and Weber's tests, was otherwise normal, and there was no past pointing, gait abnormalities, other than minimal unsteadiness, or lateralizing signs in the limbs. Romberg's test (primarily a test of the dorsal column rather than cerebellar or vestibulocochlear function) was negative. Tendon reflexes, including ankle jerks, were normal and plantar responses were downgoing bilaterally. Fundoscopy was normal. Both tympanic membranes were obscured by wax. A bedside test showed her blood sugar to be elevated, and a sample sent to the laboratory contained 18 mmol L^{-1} glucose.

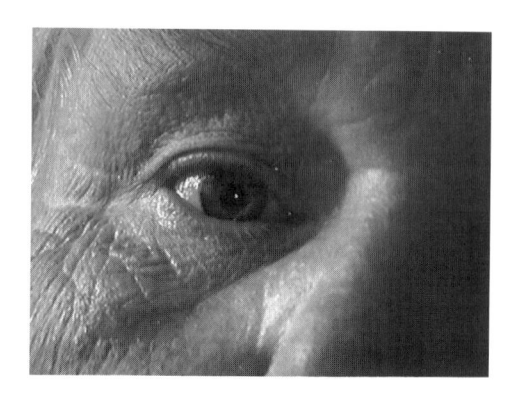

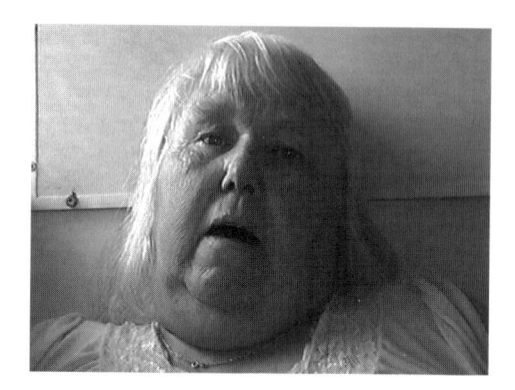

Notes

The patient had suffered a small brain stem cerebrovascular accident. The transient but nevertheless severe nausea and vomiting led to a Mallory–Weiss tear and a small haematemesis.

Basic science

Nystagmus

Nystagmus is the result of failure to maintain deviation of the eyes or postural control of eye movements. The eyes tend to drift away from the point of fixation towards the central position. Fixation is restored by a rapid, corrective flick (probably generated in the pons), the direction of which is taken as 'the direction of nystagmus'. It is usually most pronounced with maximal deviation of the eyes to one side, but may be present with the eyes in neutral position. Nystagmus on upward gaze is not 'vertical nystagmus', unless the direction of the corrective flick is itself vertical.

Optokinetic nystagmus is a normal physiological phenomenon caused by tracking movements and fast flicks (saccadic movements) to fixate on a new moving target—such as that seen in train passengers observing passing scenery. Congenital nystagmus is often familial, and consists of a steady, side to side 'wobble' of the eyes without fast flicking movements or any subjective sensation of eye movement.

Nystagmus due to disease of the VIIIth nerve, semicircular canals or the vestibular nuclei. Activation of the VIIIth nerve and vestibular apparatus pushes the eyes to the contralateral side. Any weakness in the vestibular apparatus will allow the eyes to drift back to the midline, and requires a rapid, corrective eye movement away from the side of the vestibular lesion. However, if vestibular damage develops relatively slowly, for example in Ménière's disease or VIIIth nerve damage by an acoustic neuroma, central compensation prevents nystagmus unless the brain stem is also damaged. Nystagmus following acute labyrinthine damage often resolves after an initial period, again through brain stem compensatory mechanisms.

Cerebellar nystagmus. Nystagmus is a feature of unilateral cerebellar disease. It is not a universal feature of cerebellar damage and, in some degenerative diseases and diseases affecting the midline, nystagmus may be absent despite marked ataxia in the patient. The exact mechanism of cerebellar ataxia is not known, but clinically it appears that nystagmus, if it occurs, is towards the side of the lesion.

Nystagmus caused by damage to the vestibular nuclei. The vestibular nuclei are generally damaged by vascular lesions of the brain stem or demyelination. When bilateral and associated with other lesions, complex patterns of nystagmus (ataxic nystagmus) can be produced. A midline lesion at the level of the IIIrd nerve nucleus produces a divergent strabismus (squint) with the eyes at rest, owing to the intact VIth nerves. Midline lesions at the level of the pons result in classical internuclear ophthalmoplegia with failure of adduction of each eye and marked nystagmus on abduction. Lesions at the level of the VIth nerve produce bilateral failure of abduction, with very little nystagmus on adduction.

Other causes of nystagmus. Decompensation of the brain stem by tumours or toxic effects of drugs can be vertical as well as horizontal. The fast flick, which occurs in a vertical direction, is usually seen best on upward gaze. Sedative drugs and anticonvulsants, such as phenytoin and carbamazepine, are quite commonly associated with nystagmus.

MCQs

1 Nystagmus due to vestibular and VIIIth nerve damage is usually transient.
2 Nystagmus due to vestibular and VIIIth nerve damage is away from the damaged side.
3 Nystagmus in cerebellar disease is towards the side of the lesion.
4 Ataxic nystagmus is nystagmus associated with ataxic gait.
5 Nystagmus is typically produced by vascular accidents in the middle cerebral artery territory.

Case 37
Numbness, nystagmus and a drooping eyelid

History

A 63-year-old housewife with no previous medical history was admitted to casualty with a 4-h history of loss of sensation on the left side of her body, dizziness, nausea and drooping of her right eyelid. She had retired to bed the previous evening in perfect health, as far as she knew, but woken on the morning of presentation with sensory loss on the left side which she initially attributed to 'sleeping awkwardly'. Minutes later, however, she developed severe vertigo and nausea but, by the time the patient and her husband had made their way to casualty, almost all of her symptoms had completely resolved. She ate a normal diet, drank very little alcohol, had never smoked and had no family history of diabetes mellitus, heart attacks or stroke.

The patient was anxious but otherwise looked well. Her blood pressure was 188/98 mmHg and her pulse was regular at 88 beats per minute (b.p.m.). Examination of the chest and abdomen was unremarkable. Muscle power, tendon reflexes, pinprick sensation and proprioception were symmetrical and normal. Plantar responses were downgoing and cranial nerve examination, including fundoscopy, was normal. The only abnormal finding was a right-sided Horner's syndrome, which was still evident when the patient was reviewed in the outpatient department later the same week.

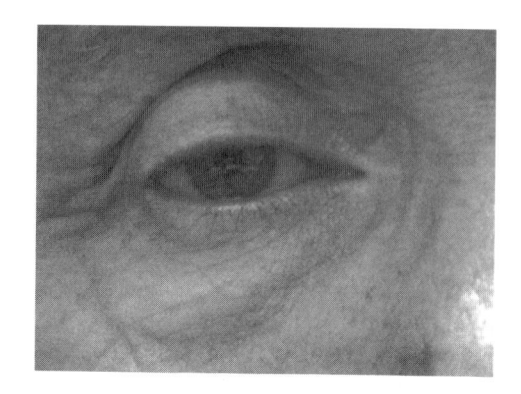

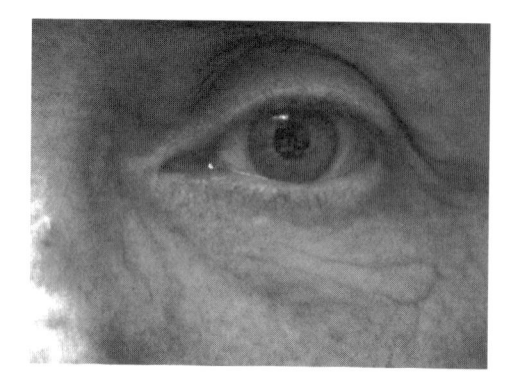

Notes

The patient had suffered a small brain stem stroke with transient ischaemia of the surrounding area, probably involving the dorsolateral region of the lower pons.

In the pons, the descending sympathetic fibres that supply the eye and the outflow from the VIIIth cranial nerve run closely together. The pons is supplied by penetrating branches of the vertebral arteries which join at the inferior border of the pons to give rise to the basilar artery. The patient was left with Horner's syndrome.

Horner's syndrome consists of pupillary constriction (miosis) and ptosis (drooping of the upper eyelid from denervation of the sympathetic nerve supply to the smooth muscle component of the levator palpebrae superioris). The signs of Horner's syndrome are often very subtle, and are best observed in low light levels as the contralateral normal pupil

patient's fasting glucose (<6.0 mmol L⁻¹) and HbA1c (4.8%) levels were within their normal ranges. She was treated with aspirin, 300 mg daily.

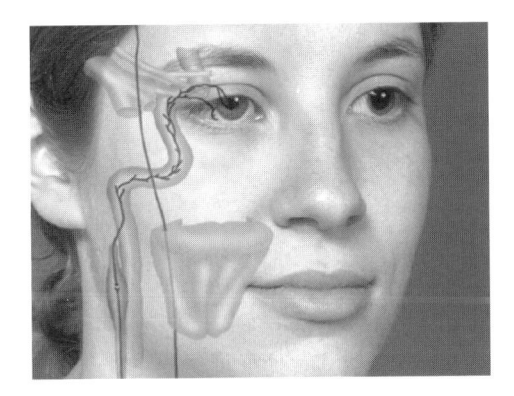

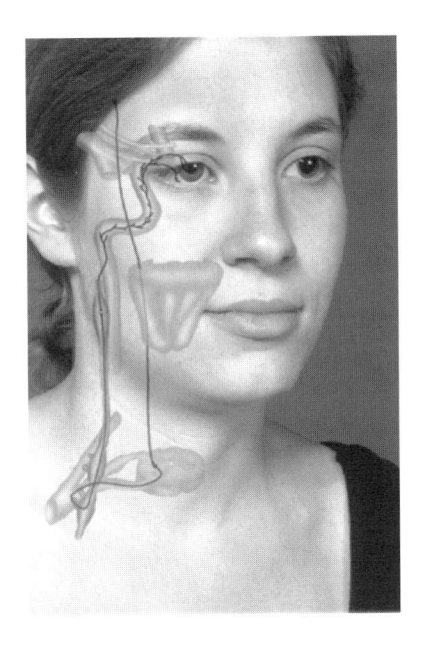

Basic science

Aspirin irreversibly acetylates and thereby inhibits platelet cyclooxygenase, which normally converts arachidonic acid to a labile endoperoxide intermediate critical for thromboxane formation. A single dose impairs haemostasis for 5–7 days. There is currently insufficient evidence to recommend the use of antiplatelet drugs in acute stroke, but their efficacy in preventing further strokes or transient ischaemic attacks is unequivocal.

Causes of Horner's syndrome

- Stroke:
    Hemisphere: a massive infarction involving the hypothalamus.
    Brain stem: a discrete lesion, particularly in the dorsolateral region.
- Other brain stem lesions:
    Tumours (i.e. gliomas and ependymomas).
    Demyelination (i.e. multiple sclerosis).
    Disruption of the brain stem (i.e. syringomyelia).
- Pancoast's syndrome:
    An apical bronchogenic neoplasm involving the T1 nerve route, which produces axillary pain, wasting of the small muscles of the hand and Horner's syndrome.
- Sympathetic chain:
    Surgery.
    Malignant disease in the neck or jugular foramen.
    Carotid aneurysm.
- T1 root damage:
    Cervical rib.
    Avulsion of the lower brachial plexus (Klumpke's paralysis).

will be dilated. The slight enophthalmos (retraction of the globe of the eye into the socket), conjunctival vasodilatation and facial hypohidrosis (reduction in sweating) that complete the syndrome are even more difficult to detect with certainty.

In the past, syphilis was the major cause of small vessel occlusion in the brain stem. Atherosclerosis, a particular problem in diabetic patients, is now the most commonly identified cause. In this patient, tests for syphilis (venereal disease research laboratory (VDRL) and *Treponema pallidum* haemagglutination (TPHA) tests) were negative, and the

MCQs

1 The presence of ptosis distinguishes Horner's syndrome from a IIIrd nerve palsy.
2 Horner's syndrome can be caused by damage to the internal capsule.
3 The signs of Horner's syndrome are best seen in bright light.
4 Ptosis in Horner's syndrome and facial nerve palsy can be distinguished by pupil size.
5 Horner's syndrome can occur in multiple sclerosis.

Case 38
The man who couldn't let go

History

A 42-year-old unemployed cinema attendant presented to casualty having stumbled over an uneven paving slab in the street. Although in no pain, he found that, quite unexpectedly, he had been unable to get up without help. The people who stopped to help him called an ambulance, and he was seen in accident and emergency. The 'trouble' had apparently started 5 years previously when he had been walking along with his then enormously obese wife on his arm. He tripped and was unfortunate enough to pull her down on top of him. They had to take a taxi home and, from that time on, he had suffered a gradual and inexplicable physical and social decline, having last worked as a cinema attendant 2 years previously. The only potentially significant family history was of a cousin who died in his fifth decade of unknown cause, and another cousin on his paternal side who was said to have 'a drooping eyelid'.

On examination, the patient was haggard and unkempt, but able to give a clear account of the injury that led to his admission to hospital. There were no abnormal findings on examination of his chest or abdomen, but his testes were noted to be small and soft. He had marked temporal recession and mild bilateral ptosis. Sensation was normal, but muscle power was globally reduced, with marked weakness and wasting of his sternomastoid muscles. Fundoscopy was normal, but percussion of his thenar eminences produced an abnormal response.

Notes

The patient had myotonic dystrophy.

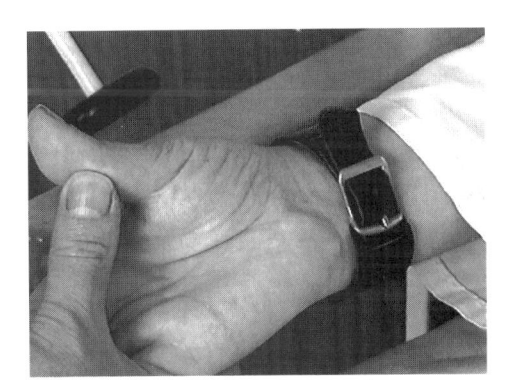

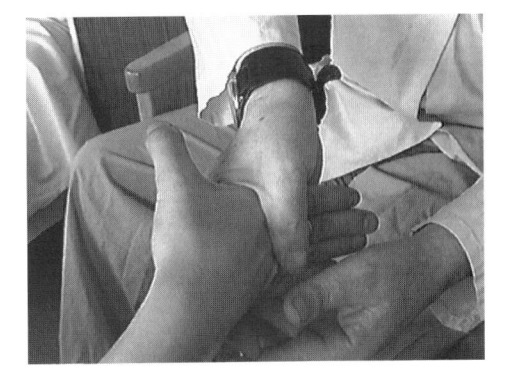

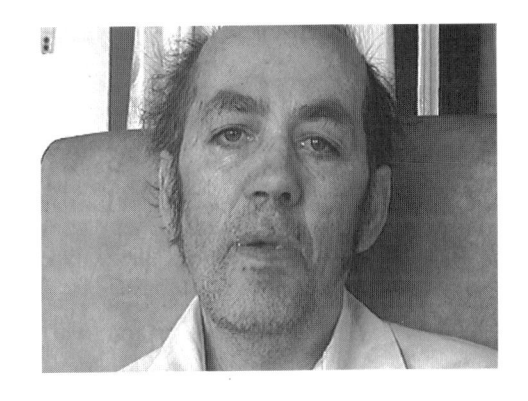

Myotonic dystrophy (Steinert's disease) is an autosomal dominant condition that usually manifests in young adulthood. It is the most common adult myopathy, with a prevalence of around 50 per million of the population. The presence of isolated signs in other family members suggests that disease penetrance is variable. The most striking manifestation is myotonia. In this case, the patient had particular difficulty lifting items off shelves, because he had to grip hard to do so and was then unable to put the objects down. Paradoxically, marked muscle wasting and weakness is also associated, one of the most conspicuously affected muscle groups being the sternocleidomastoids. Numerous other associated features include mental slowing, cataracts, frontal balding, ptosis and testicular atrophy.

Basic science

Trinucleotide repeat expansions

The mutation underlying myotonic dystrophy is caused by a trinucleotide repeat expansion (CTG)n, located in the 3′ untranslated region of the dystrophia myotonica protein kinase gene. The cellular effects of the CTG expansion and how it leads to the diverse, multisystem clinical phenotype of myotonic dystrophy are unknown.

Expansion of repeating triplets of nucleotides in the genome has recently been associated with nine degenerative and developmental neuropsychiatric diseases: fragile X syndrome, fragile X-linked mental retardation, myotonic dystrophy, Friedreich's ataxia, spinal and bulbar muscular atrophy, Huntington's disease, spinocerebellar ataxia type 1, dentatorubral-pallidoluysian atrophy and Machado–Joseph disease. These diseases are all conditions of the central nervous system. In all of them, the inheritance pattern usually exhibits the phenomenon of anticipation (defined as progressively earlier age of onset or a worsening disease severity over successive generations). The severity of the phenotypic expression and penetrance appears to be related to the extent of the triplet expansion.

Myotonic syndromes (in addition to myotonic dystrophy)

Myotonia congenita (Thomsen's disease). This is an autosomal dominant condition produced by a defect in the gene coding for a muscle chloride channel located at 7q35. Myotonia is usually present in childhood and persists throughout life, but the presentation of myotonia congenita differs considerably even within families. Warm up exercises decrease myotonia, and the strength of the hypertrophied muscles is normal or even enhanced.

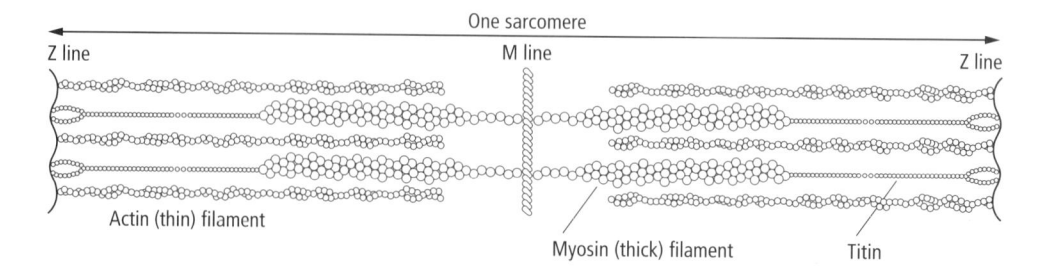

Myotonia congenita (Becker's disease). Becker's disease is again the result of an abnormal muscle chloride channel gene, but the inheritance is autosomal recessive. Clinical features are myotonia, usually more severe than that seen in Thomsen's disease, that manifests in childhood or the early teenage years and persists throughout life. The strength of the hypertrophied muscles is again normal, but tends to decrease on exercise, even though myotonia also decreases with warm up exercises. The neck, shoulder and arm muscles are usually atrophic.

Other forms of myotonia. Myotonia fluctuans is an autosomal dominant condition caused by mutation of a muscle sodium channel subunit. Myotonia is precipitated by exercise, develops during rest within 30 min and lasts for about 1 h. The condition is worsened by potassium loading and depolarizing muscle relaxants, such as suxamethonium, but is unaffected by the cold.

Paramyotonia congenita is an autosomal dominant condition caused by a similar mutation to that in myotonia fluctuans. The myotonia is markedly exacerbated by the cold.

Chondrodystrophic myotonia (Schwartz–Jampel syndrome) is an autosomal recessive condition presenting within the first 3 years of life, characterized by multiple skeletal deformities, myopia and small stature. Thigh muscles are hypertrophic and shoulder muscles atrophic.

MCQs

1 The stiffness in myotonic dystrophy and myotonia congenita tends to improve with 'warm up'.
2 Myotonic dystrophy is inherited as an autosomal dominant condition.
3 The characteristic feature of myotonic dystrophy is myotonia in the presence of muscle wasting and weakness.
4 Myotonic dystrophy is associated with hypogonadism.
5 Frontal balding, ptosis and dislocation of the lens are associated with myotonic dystrophy.

Case 39
Ear pain and facial weakness

History

A 78-year-old housewife was admitted with a 2-day history of severe pain in the right ear and disturbance of balance. This was followed 24h later by the appearance of a vesicular rash around the ear and fauces, and by the development of mild right-sided facial weakness.

On examination, a crusted rash was present in the external auditory meatus and inner part of the auricle (the concha and antitragus). Close inspection revealed weakness of the right side of the face affecting all areas including the forehead. There were no other significant related findings.

Notes

The patient had developed Ramsay–Hunt syndrome.

Ramsay–Hunt syndrome is caused by herpes zoster infection of the VIIth cranial nerve (geniculate ganglion). The patient often experiences severe pain in the ear and/or throat, followed by facial palsy and sometimes by deafness and vertigo. When the geniculate ganglion of the facial nerve is involved, the VIIth nerve sensory innervation of the palate and fauces via the greater petrosal nerve and the auricle carried on the auricular branch of the Xth nerve are affected. General oedema around the nerve causes lower motor neurone motor weakness affecting all of the ipsilateral muscles of facial expression, hence the facial weakness involving the forehead. Full recovery of facial nerve function after herpes zoster infection is less likely than recovery after idiopathic lower motor neurone VIIth nerve palsy (Bell's palsy), in which 60% recover completely.

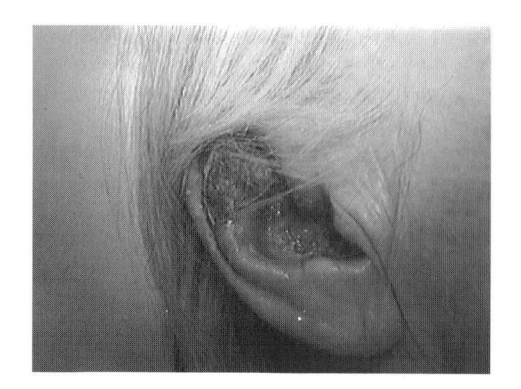

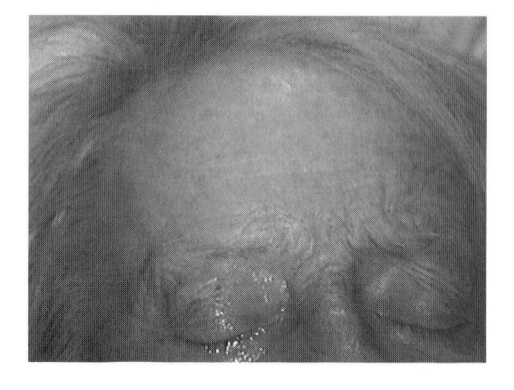

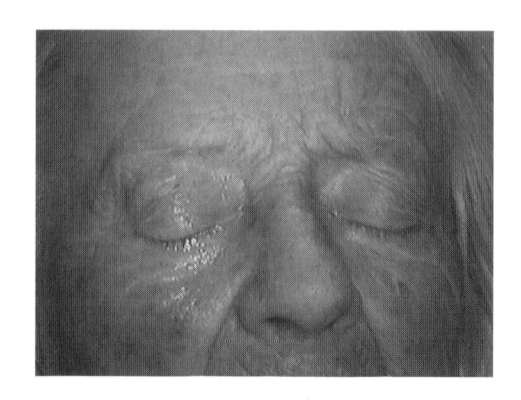

Basic science

Chicken pox (varicella) and shingles are different manifestations of infection with the herpes zoster virus. In shingles, herpes zoster infection produces a sensory neuritis characterized by acute inflammation of one or more posterior root ganglia, spinal nerves or roots and grey matter of the spinal cord. Herpes zoster is mainly a disease of adults, in whom the virus has remained dormant in spinal ganglia since an episode of chicken pox many years previously. As the vesicles contain intact virus particles, intimate contact with a patient with herpes zoster can give rise to chicken pox in a susceptible individual. The development of shingles after exposure to chicken pox is much rarer and is thought to be due to reinfection-induced reactivation in a patient who has already been exposed to chicken pox. Neoplasms, such as Hodgkin's disease, that are associated with the impairment of cell-mediated immunity are frequently associated with the reactivation of herpes zoster. Recurrent herpes zoster infection is thought to be very unusual. The thorax is involved in 55% of cases, the neck in 20% and the lumbar and sacral nerves in 15%.

Pain referred to the ear

When examination of the ear fails to reveal any pathology, the diagnosis and management of otalgia can encompass the fields of oral surgery and dentistry, neurology and neurosurgery, as well as general medicine and ear, nose and throat (ENT) medicine. The following causes of ear pain are worth considering:
- Chronic sinusitis. Patients with chronic sinusitis classically present with several weeks of headaches and fatigue, facial and ear pain, pressure between the eyes, nasal congestion and a postnasal drip. The headache is often worse in the morning, and tends to be exacerbated by head movement.
- Temporomandibular joint disorder. Tinnitus, vertigo and other symptoms referred to the ear, including pain (in 48%), are known to occur in association with temporomandibular joint disorder. A similar proportion of patients with temporomandibular joint disorder complain of headache, sinus pain or neck pain. The mechanism of the association of temporomandibular joint disorder and otologic symptoms is unknown.
- Chest infections. Pneumonia caused by atypical organisms usually has extrapulmonary features. Mycoplasmal pneumonia, in particular, may manifest with ear pain and a non-productive cough.
- Gastro-oesophageal reflux. There is some evidence that, in young children, pain derived from gastro-oesophageal reflux may be referred to the ear. Fretful, irritable children who pull on their ears and present with what is thought to be recurrent otitis media, but have normal tympanic membranes, may be better treated with an anti-reflux regimen.
- Cervicogenic otalgia. Ear pain referred from the cervical spine, 'cervicogenic otalgia', is thought to be responsible for about 6% of cases presenting with ear pain.
- Migraine. A proportion of migraine sufferers have pain referred to the ear or a feeling of aural fullness, sometimes associated with intermittent vestibular symptoms.
- Others. In addition to psychogenic otalgia, referred otalgia may also be caused by neoplasms, dental abnormalities or infections, pharyngeal or salivary gland infections, temporal arteritis or one of the neuralgias.

MCQs

1 Contact of a susceptible individual with a person with shingles can lead to chicken pox.
2 Gastro-oesophageal reflux can present as recurrent otitis in young children.

3 Herpes viruses are DNA viruses.
4 Varicella pneumonitis is a rare complication of chicken pox in adults.
5 Ramsay–Hunt syndrome results when the ciliary ganglion of the IIIrd nerve is involved.

Case 40
Muscle weakness and wasting

History

A 74-year-old retired draughtsman was seen in clinic with a long history of muscular wasting and weakness that had started in his childhood. He had first come to medical attention at the age of 12 years, when he presented with painful feet which were, to use his own description, 'a little bit twisted'. He also complained of muscular weakness in his legs (i.e. below the knee), but at that time had no problem with weakness of his arms, forearms or hands, although he was told that the condition would be likely to affect his upper limbs with time and would gradually worsen in his legs. The wasting of his leg muscles gradually developed throughout his childhood, and showed considerable wasting by the time he was 20 years old. His advisers at the time suggested that he opted for a career in which he would 'keep his hands working'. Eventually, by the age of 53 years, he found that he was unable to continue his career as a draughtsman and retired from work. The weakness at the time not only prevented him from working but also, for example, prevented him from being able to pick up a small object, such as a screw, from the ground if he dropped it in the garage.

On examination, there was marked wasting of the peroneal muscles of both legs. He had undergone surgery to his left ankle to correct valgus deformity at that level, and a number of hammer toes (one on the right and two on the left) had been amputated. All of his hand muscles were markedly wasted.

Notes

The patient had peroneal muscular atrophy.
Charcot–Marie–Tooth disease (type 1A) is the most common inherited disorder of the

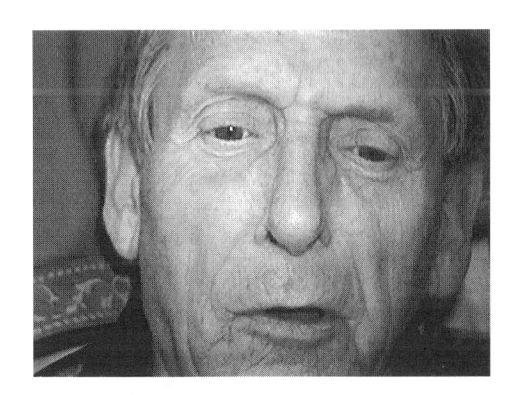

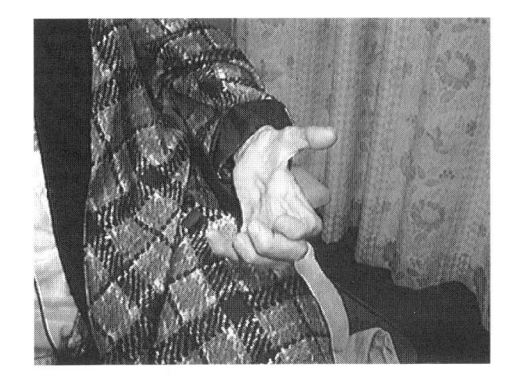

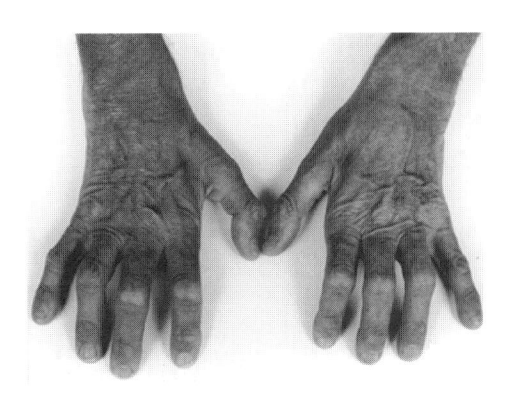

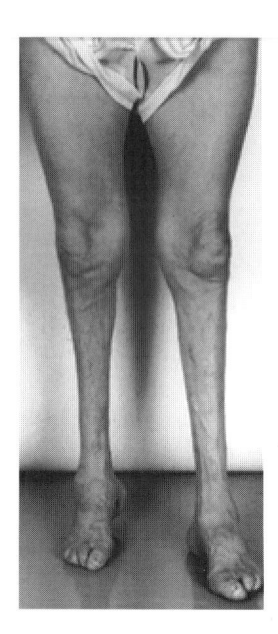

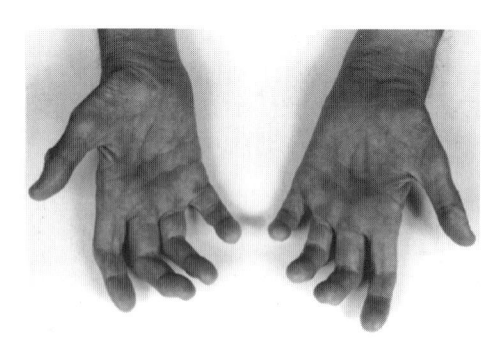

peripheral nervous system. It is an autosomal dominant demyelinating polyneuropathy which results from duplications or point mutations of the gene for 'peripheral myelin protein 22' on chromosome 17p11.2-p12. Deletion of the same portion of chromosome 17 gives rise to 'hereditary neuropathy with liability to pressure palsies'.

Charcot–Marie–Tooth disease usually manifests between infancy (with delayed ability to walk) and the second decade of life (with often marked proximal muscle weakness of the lower extremities). The clinical phenotypes, which include foot deformity, progressive distal muscle atrophy and weakness, gait abnormalities, absent reflexes, sensory impairment and invariable symmetric reductions in motor nerve conduction velocities on electrophysiologic testing, are extremely variable in severity. Nevertheless, individuals remain ambulatory and there is no decrease in lifespan.

Basic science

Peripheral neuropathy

Relatively common causes of peripheral neuropathy include diabetes mellitus and carcinomatous neuropathy. Thiamine deficiency, vitamin B_{12} deficiency and the effects of drugs and chemicals are less commonly seen, and polyarteritis nodosa, Guillain–Barré syndrome, amyloidosis, sarcoidosis, brachial neuritis and porphyria are rarer still.

An underlying carcinoma is an important differential diagnosis in peripheral neuropathy. Direct compression or infiltration of spinal roots or peripheral or cranial nerve trunks or branches can be identified easily when they occur in established malignancy, but may be more difficult to diagnose when they are presenting features.

In paraneoplastic sensory neuropathy, autoantibodies to neuronal antigens have become useful diagnostic markers for an underlying carcinoma, especially anti-Hu antibodies. Strong circumstantial evidence suggests that the autoimmune response that leads to the formation of these antibodies may be responsible for the pathogenesis of some of these neuropathic syndromes. Neuropathy appearing during the course of treatment of carcinoma may be due to radiation-induced damage or the neurotoxic effects of some chemotherapeutic agents.

Guillain–Barré syndrome is a heterogeneous disorder in terms of clinical characteristics, course, prognosis and underlying pathology.

A better understanding of the principal mechanisms of autoimmunity in the peripheral nervous system will aid the development of more specific and efficacious treatments.

MCQs

1 Sensory impairment is a feature of peroneal muscular atrophy.
2 Charcot–Marie–Tooth disease is an autosomal dominant condition.
3 Malignancy-related sensory neuropathy is likely to be mediated by an immune mechanism.
4 Symptoms and signs of Charcot–Marie–Tooth disease may develop in infancy.
5 Charcot–Marie–Tooth disease usually results in a decrease in lifespan.

Case 41
Table tennis was fine

History

A 45-year-old tax inspector was admitted via accident and emergency with a 2-day history of increasing difficulty finding words. A few days before his admission, he had been playing table tennis with friends and, with no previous history of illness of any kind, considered himself to be completely well. His wife, in retrospect, had noted that for the previous 6 weeks or perhaps longer he had occasionally stumbled over words or answered inappropriately, but she too had not been unduly concerned at the time. He denied any problems with muscle weakness or headaches and had suffered no visual impairment. His alcohol intake was modest. He had smoked 5–10 cigars daily since his late teenage years.

On examination, his speech was characterized by entirely normal comprehension and only minimally impaired ability to read and write, but almost complete inability to find appropriate words. Cranial nerve examination was normal. The only other finding was bilateral papilloedema, more marked on the left than the right, with haemorrhages around the optic disc. There were no other lateralizing or localizing signs of neurological disease, and examination of the chest and abdomen was entirely unremarkable. His blood pressure was 144/86 mmHg. An urgent CT scan of his head was carried out with and without intravenous contrast enhancement.

Notes

The patient was found to have a giant aneurysm, partly filled with clot, in the lower temporal area on the left side.

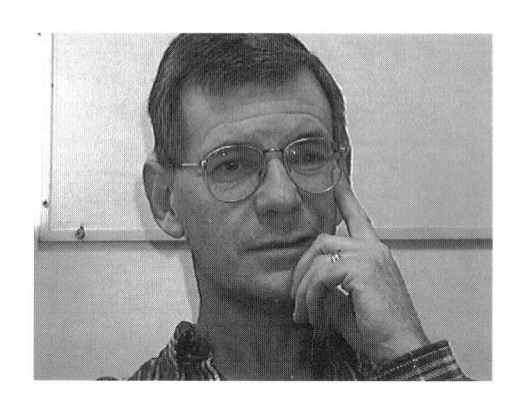

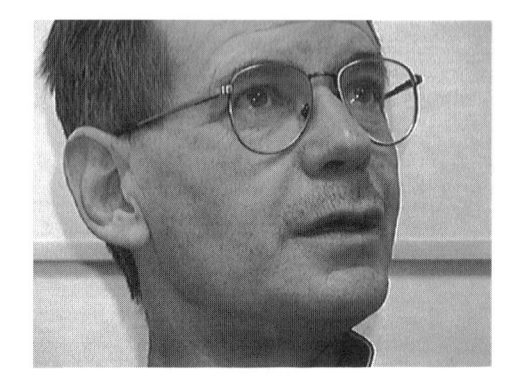

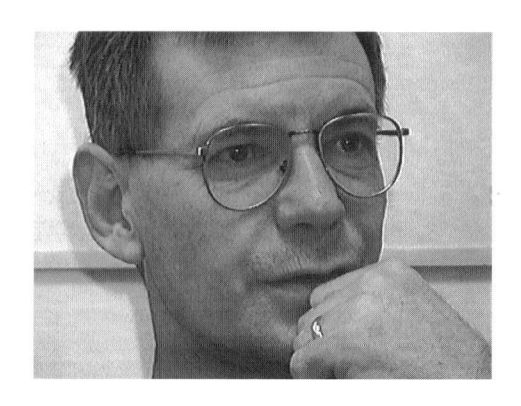

The increasingly rapid expansion of this and the surrounding oedema it induced had obstructed cerebrospinal fluid outflow causing raised intracranial pressure and papilloedema. Involvement of the temporal and lower pole of the frontal lobe (Broca's motor speech area) was responsible for his unusual presentation with motor dysphasia.

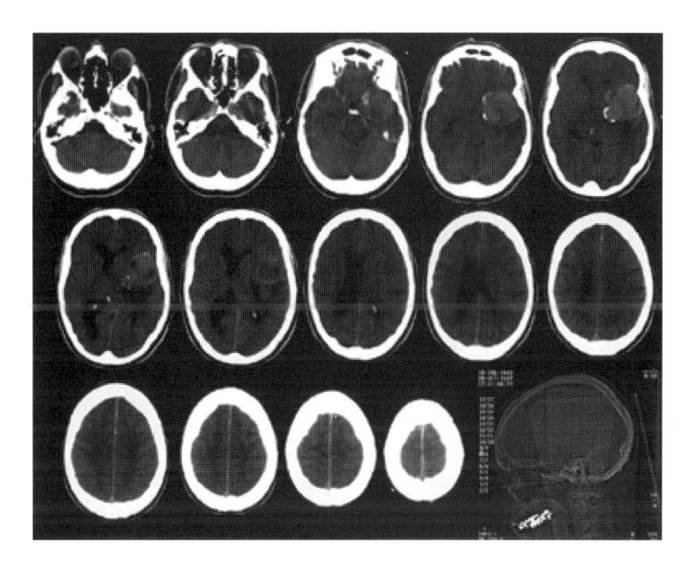

Aneurysms more than 2 cm in diameter tend to occur at the same sites as smaller aneurysms. When localized distal to the bifurcations of the great vessels and the circle of Willis, however, an infective (mycotic) aneurysm, sometimes the result of showers of infected emboli from bacterial endocarditis, is more likely. Whether infective or not, as major brain compression and death occur if giant aneurysms are left untreated, neurosurgical decompression is the primary therapy.

Basic science

Intracranial haemorrhage

There are many causes of intracranial haemorrhage, including, for example, trauma and bleeding disorders, haemorrhage into a region of cerebral infarction and hypertensive haemorrhage, which can often be shown to have arisen from one of the arteries of the circle of Willis or one of the penetrating (lenticulostriate) branches of the middle cerebral artery. The most common spontaneous causes of intracranial haemorrhage are ruptured saccular aneurysms and bleeding from arteriovenous malformations. The blood tends to dissect rapidly through adjacent brain tissue over a period of a few minutes, but does not usually rupture through the grey matter of the cortical surface. With large haemorrhages, the patient rapidly lapses into coma, but, more often, typical lateralizing signs of facial and limb weakness appear and progress to complete flaccid hemiplegia over a period of up to 30 min.

In pontine haemorrhages, deep coma rapidly occurs in association with pinpoint pupils, impairment of doll's eyes movements, hypertension and frequently hyperpyrexia, leading to death within a few hours.

Autopsy series have shown that saccular aneurysms occur in 5% of the population at large. In up to 30%, multiple aneurysms are present. They are usually found at the bifurcations of large arteries at the base of the brain, particularly the junction of the posterior communicating artery and the internal carotid artery and the junction of the anterior communicating and anterior cerebral arteries. The annual risk of rupture is 1 : 25 000. Approximately 25% of patients who rupture a saccular aneurysm die within 24 h, and the death rate at 3 months is almost 50%. Of the remaining patients, more than 50% are left with major neurological impairment.

MCQs

1 Rupture of a saccular aneurysm is the most common cause of spontaneous intracranial haemorrhage.
2 Saccular aneurysms occur in 5% of the population.
3 The death rate from a ruptured berry aneurysm at 3 months is 25%.
4 Of those who survive a ruptured berry aneurysm, 50% are left with major neurological impairment.
5 Pontine haemorrhage is typically associated with pupillary dilatation.

Case 42
The smell that wasn't there

History

A 24-year-old researcher for a company that made natural history films was admitted to hospital after a fit. His history started just over a year previously, when he presented to his GP with a persistent cough accompanied by breathlessness. Despite a course of antibiotics and stopping smoking, his symptoms persisted, and he was sent for a chest X-ray. On the basis of the radiographic findings, he was referred to the respiratory physicians who carried out a mediastinoscopy to obtain lymph node biopsies. Some months after his original presentation, he noticed a lump above his right eye and also noticed marked deterioration in vision severe enough to prevent him from reading. He attended the casualty department of the eye hospital, where a diagnosis of anterior uveitis was made. Subsequently, he developed nocturia, occurring at intervals throughout the night, and thirst. On the day of admission, he had been walking in town when he noticed a vague sensation and an unusual, but not unpleasant, smell that persisted for 2 h. A similar event happened at home, and a third much more severe episode while he was ascending the stairs. The next thing he knew he was at the bottom of the stairs with paramedics standing over him. He had bitten his tongue and cracked a vertebra on his way down the stairs. A magnetic resonance imaging (MRI) scan was requested in hospital

Notes

The fits and diabetes insipidus were manifestations of cerebral sarcoidosis.

The lymph node biopsy confirmed the diagnosis of pulmonary sarcoidosis and, in addition to sarcoid-induced anterior uveitis complicated by glaucoma, the patient developed cerebral sarcoidosis with partial complex seizures characterized by an olfactory aura (an uncinate fit). Involvement of the temporal lobes and diffuse involvement of the hypothalamus were likely to have been the causative lesions for the olfactory hallucination and seizure, and the diabetes insipidus, respectively.

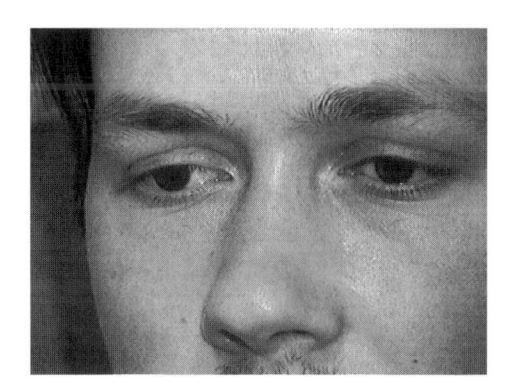

All components of the nervous system can be affected by sarcoidosis, and the incidence of cerebral involvement in cases of sarcoidosis is between 1.7 and 3.5%. Unilateral, transient involvement of the facial nerve is relatively common, and the most usual pattern seen on MRI scan is diffuse involvement of the periventricular white matter with multifocal involvement of the cerebral white matter. Diffuse meningeal involvement is sometimes seen with contrast-enhanced CT scanning. Cranial and peripheral nerve involvement can occur, as can the formation of a space-occupying lesion, but, although the clinical course is unpredictable, the prognosis is generally favourable.

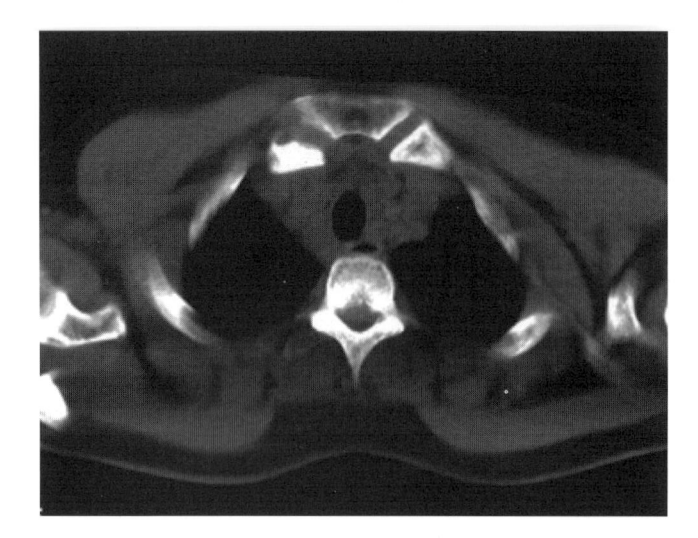

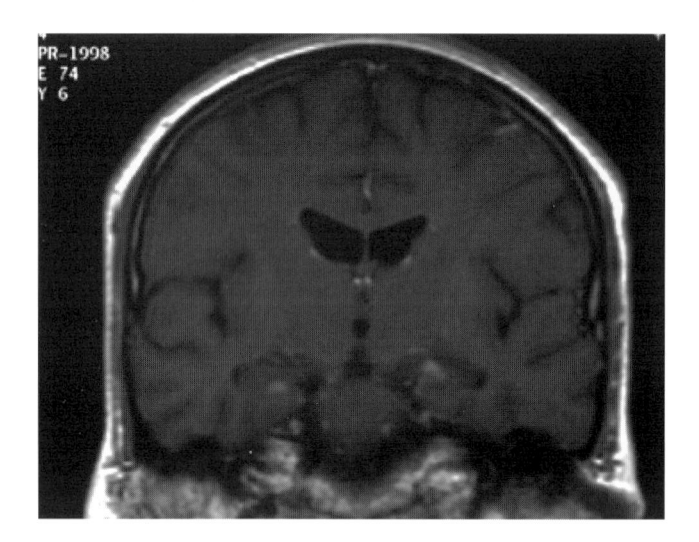

Basic science

Olfaction

The olfactory system, the rhinencephalon or nosebrain, dominates the cerebral hemispheres of lower vertebrates. In humans, the system consists of the olfactory nerve cells in the olfactory mucosa in the nose, which covers an area of about 5 cm² in total. The nerve filaments project through the foramina in the cribriform plate of the ethmoid bone at the base of the anterior cranial fossa to the olfactory bulb. The olfactory bulb is connected to the brain by the olfactory tract, a strip of palaeocortex extending anteriorly from the uncus of the temporal lobe. The rhinencephalon itself has become incorporated into the hippocampus and dentate gyrus of the temporal lobe as part of the limbic system. The sense of smell in humans is less important than most other senses, but still contributes

tants, have recently been shown unequivocally to exist in humans. The synchronization of menstrual cycles of women who sleep in the same dormitory is a manifestation of the same phenomenon.

MCQs

1 Cerebral sarcoidosis does not involve the spinal cord.
2 Multifocal involvement of the cerebral hemispheres can produce diabetes insipidus.
3 Bilateral, chronic facial nerve palsies are characteristic of sarcoidosis.
4 An olfactory aura preceding a fit suggests involvement of the frontal lobes.
5 Cranial sarcoidosis can present as a space-occupying lesion.

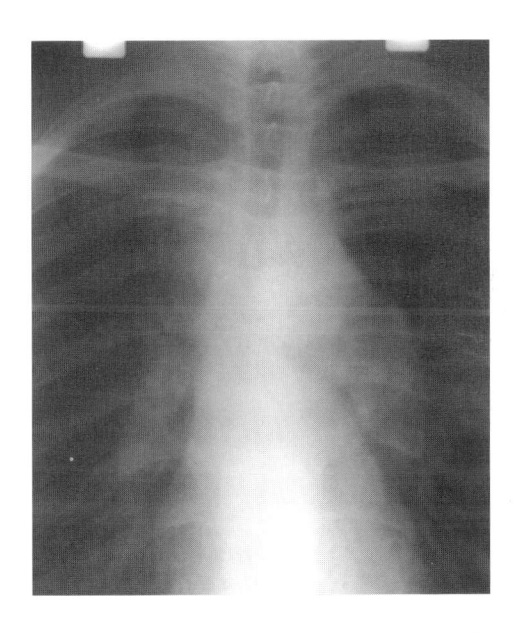

significantly to the pleasure of eating and can conjure up memories and emotions. Pheromones, chemicals which both modify gonadal axis function and act as sexual attrac-

Case 43
Breathlessness after a road traffic accident

History

A 49-year-old telephonist was admitted to hospital with a long history of shortness of breath. The history started after a road traffic accident, in which she sustained a severe fracture of her left leg which required fixation and a prolonged period of recovery in hospital. She noted some shortness of breath particularly on waking in the morning, despite being confined to bed, but did not complain of the symptom at the time. When she was eventually discharged from hospital, she realized that even minimal exertion resulted in marked breathlessness. She duly mentioned the problem when she was next seen in the orthopaedic outpatient department, and was referred for a respiratory opinion. Reduced air entry and widespread crackles were heard on auscultation of both lung fields. There was no finger clubbing, no lymphadenopathy and no evidence of carbon dioxide retention. Her respiratory rate at rest was slightly increased. A chest X-ray was carried out. Blood tests, which included a full blood count, urea and electrolytes, calcium and phosphate, were normal.

The chest X-ray showed widespread interstitial opacification throughout both lungs. There was more linear opacification in both upper zones, with marked upper zone volume loss, and multiple small calcific opacities over both hila, suggesting old tuberculous granulomas. There was some evidence of a reduction in volume of the right middle and lower lobes.

Notes

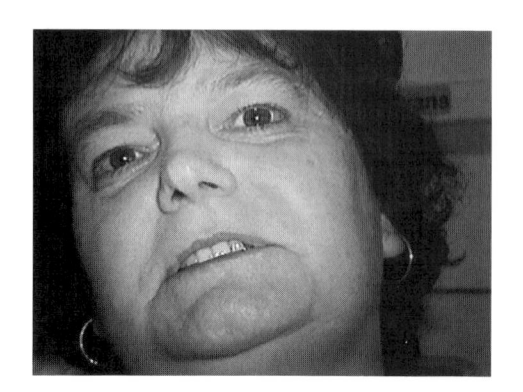

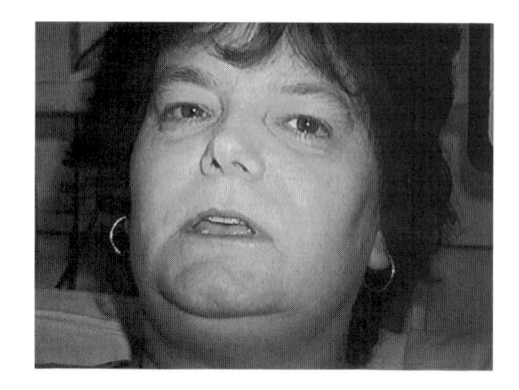

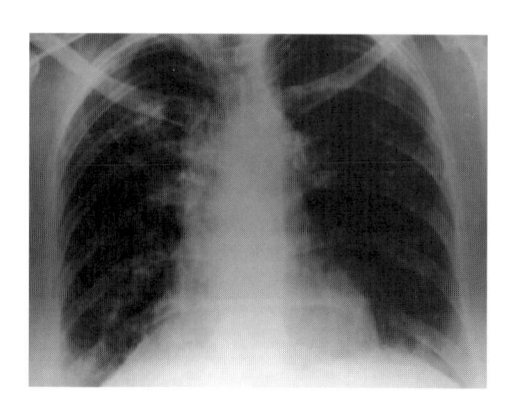

The patient had pulmonary fibrosis from pulmonary sarcoidosis (diagnosed histologically after bronchoscopy). This was one of the patient's many hospital admissions with exacerbation of breathlessness.

Sarcoidosis is a multisystem granulomatous disease of unknown aetiology characterized by the formation of widespread non-caseating epithelioid cell granulomas. The most frequent and benign presentation is with bilateral hilar lymphadenopathy and erythema nodosum. Pulmonary infiltration, skin and eye lesions, peripheral lymph node involvement and involvement of the liver, spleen, mucous membranes, parotid glands, phalangeal bones, muscles, heart and nervous system are well described. Approximately 50% of patients with pulmonary sarcoidosis develop permanent pulmonary abnormalities, and up to 20% have the progressive pulmonary fibrosis seen in this case. Pulmonary lymphadenopathy is present in 75–90% of patients with pulmonary sarcoidosis.

The prevalence of the condition is 10–40:100 000. All peoples are affected, but American blacks are affected 10 times more frequently than whites. There is characteristically impairment of cell-mediated immunity (manifested by the absence of a response to tuberculin), and corticosteroids are often used successfully to produce clinical remissions and to suppress inflammation and granuloma formation.

Basic science

Pathogenesis of sarcoid granulomas

In sarcoidosis, recent research suggests that local antigen-driven immune responses result in the expansion of oligoclonal populations of T cells at sites of inflammation. The expression of cytokines, such as interferon-γ and interleukin-12, dominates tissue inflammation, and the accumulation of T-helper type 1 (Th-1) cells (from which these cytokines are derived) is thought to be central to the development of granulomatous responses and to the remodelling of tissue surrounding granulomas, in keeping with experimental models of such diseases. The production of cytokines, as part of an exaggerated host immunological response, is thought to be a major contributor to lung damage and subsequent fibrosis.

The incidental finding of granulomas in liver biopsy specimens is not unusual. Around 4% of all liver biopsy specimens contain granulomas and, of these, one in seven are caused by sarcoidosis. In the lung, the diffuse pattern of sarcoidosis involvement can be difficult to distinguish from the adverse effects of cytotoxics and immunosuppressive agents (such as cyclophosphamide and D-penicillamine), silicosis, autoimmune alveolitis and idiopathic fibrosing alveolitis.

MCQs

1 Pneumothorax and wheezing are common complications of pulmonary sarcoidosis.
2 An inhaled pathogen has been implicated in pulmonary sarcoidosis.
3 The most common organs to be involved clinically with sarcoidosis are the lungs, skin, eyes and lymph nodes.
4 Cytokines produced by Th-1 lymphocytes are implicated in the pathogenesis of granulomatous tissue reactions.
5 Granulomas are found incidentally in almost 1 in 20 liver biopsies.

Case 44
Progressive breathlessness

History

A 55-year-old plasterer, who had spent almost the whole of his working life in the building trade, began to notice that he became unusually short of breath when exerting himself. He thought that the symptoms might relate to a chest infection, and he duly gave up smoking cigarettes, which he had consumed at the rate of 20 per day since the age of 15 years. He was made redundant from his job and, soon afterwards, suffered an attack of bronchitis which was treated by his GP with a course of antibiotics. At the same time, he began to notice that his fingernails and toenails had changed shape remarkably, and that his fingers had 'thickened at the ends'. The GP was not happy with the recovery he made from the chest infection, and requested a chest X-ray before referring him for further investigations in hospital. Subsequently, he was treated with a course of steroids and azathioprine, but his breathlessness gradually progressed and he began to find it difficult to ascend stairs. He had no significant past medical history, but had almost certainly been exposed to asbestos during his career in the building industry.

On examination, he was moderately tachypnoeic at rest, with widespread inspiratory and expiratory crackles heard throughout both lung fields on auscultation. He was noted to have marked finger clubbing and mild peripheral oedema bilaterally.

Notes

The patient had idiopathic fibrosing alveolitis.

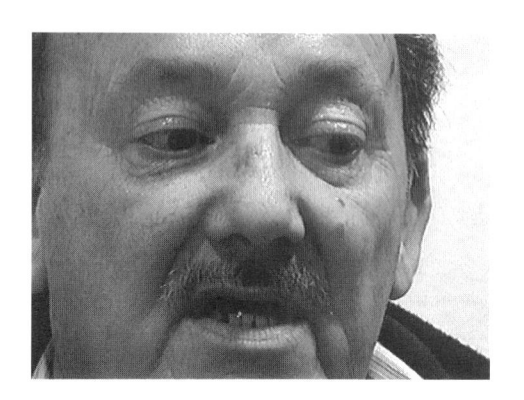

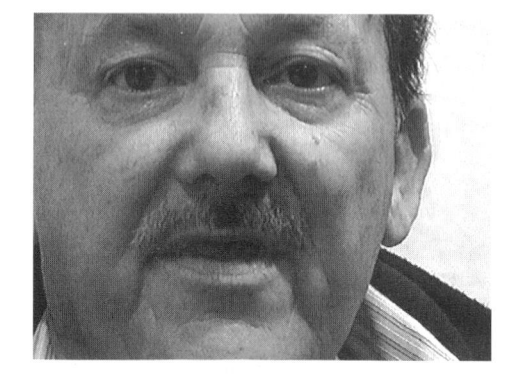

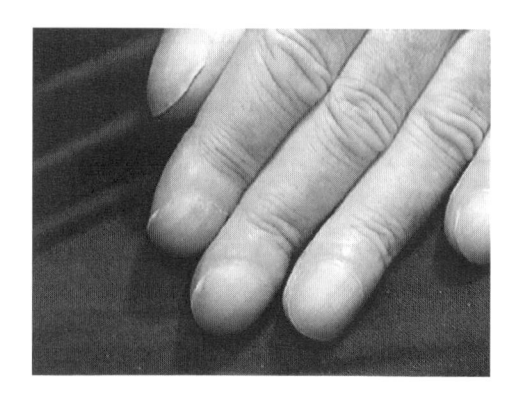

Idiopathic fibrosing alveolitis is characterized symptomatically by unremitting and progressive breathlessness, usually in middle age or the elderly, commonly associated with marked finger clubbing. It is a generally fatal disorder, with a reported median survival of 3–6 years and an estimated 10-year survival of around 27%. The mechanisms that control the progression from potentially reversible fibrogenesis to irreversible fibrosis remain unknown.

The functional abnormality is a classical restrictive pattern with a decrease in vital capacity, but a normal forced expiratory volume in 1 s to forced vital capacity (FEV1/FVC) ratio. Total lung capacity is reduced without a change in residual capacity. The most consistent early change is a reduction in the diffusing capacity of the lungs, with a reduction in P_aO_2 on exercise and eventually at rest, due to the shunting of blood to underventilated areas of the lung and to thickening of the alveolar membrane.

These changes are associated with hyperpnoea which, in the early stages of the condition, reduces P_aCO_2 and with decreased lung compliance, which increases the work of breathing and leads to the subjective sense of dyspnoea.

The principal histological features of fibrosing alveolitis are cellular thickening of the alveolar walls (with a mixed infiltrate of lymphocytes, plasma cells, giant cells, mononuclear cells and eosinophils), a tendency to fibrosis and the presence of large mononuclear cells within the alveolar spaces that have desquamated from the alveolar walls.

The differential diagnosis of idiopathic fibrosing alveolitis includes rheumatoid disease, systemic sclerosis, Sjögren's syndrome and coeliac disease. Pulmonary fibrosis also occurs as a side-effect of certain drugs, such as busulfan, bleomycin and methotrexate.

Basic science

Gas exchange

External respiration is the absorption of oxygen and excretion of carbon dioxide from the body. Internal respiration is the exchange of gas between cells and cell fluid. At rest, 12–15 breaths per minute move 6–8 L of air into and out of the airways. The air mixes with alveolar gas and, by simple diffusion through a fine layer of surfactant produced by type II pneumocytes and through an epithelium of type I pneumocytes and capillary endothelium separated by a basement membrane, 250 mL of oxygen enters red cells passing through pulmonary capillaries and 200 mL of carbon dioxide is excreted.

Normal airflow with each breath moves the 'tidal volume'. Of this, ≈150 mL fills the anatomical 'dead space'—conducting airways between the mouth and respiratory bronchioles that have no gas exchange capability. At the end of a quiet expiration, the air remaining within the lungs is the 'functional residual capacity', a proportion of which can be exhaled by a conscious exhalatory effort. The air that remains in the lung after a full expiratory effort is the margin that makes the 'total lung capacity' bigger than the 'vital capacity', which is the maximum volume that can be exhaled after a full inspiratory effort.

MCQs

1 Normal airflow with each breath is measured as the total lung capacity.
2 The volume of air in conducting airways that have no gas exchange capability constitutes the 'functional residual capacity'.
3 Air contains 21% oxygen and 4% carbon dioxide.
4 The normal resting respiratory rate is 6–10 breaths per minute.
5 Fibrosing alveolitis produces a classical restrictive pattern of pulmonary function.

Case 45
A rash and stiff hands

History

A 55-year-old businessman was seen in clinic with a 12-year history of an erythematous, scaly skin rash sparing his face, but otherwise affecting his whole body at various times. The rash responded well but transiently to psoralen therapy plus UVA radiation (PUVA) treatment and dithranol cream. Over the last 5 years, he had noticed some stiffness in his hands and feet, particularly in the morning, and observed the gradual development of painless deformities to the extent that he now found it difficult to pick up a pencil or dress himself. Current treatment with methotrexate had reduced the rash on his body and limbs, but had produced very little effect on the lesions on his hands and forearms. He had no family history of skin diseases as far as he knew. Serology revealed that he was rheumatoid factor negative. His serum urate level was $0.2\,\text{mmol}\,L^{-1}$ (normal range = 0.12–$0.42\,\text{mmol}\,L^{-1}$).

Notes

The patient had arthritis mutilans, a form of psoriatic arthritis.

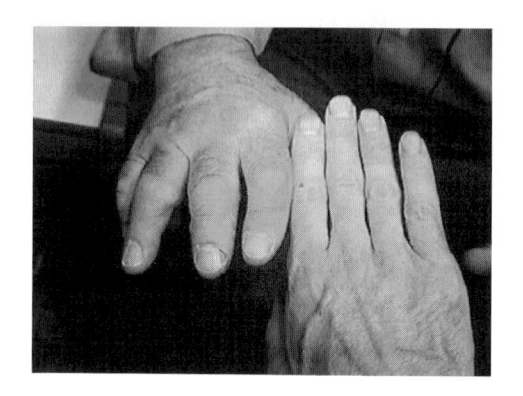

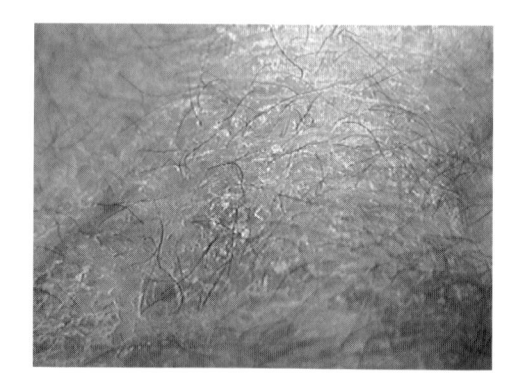

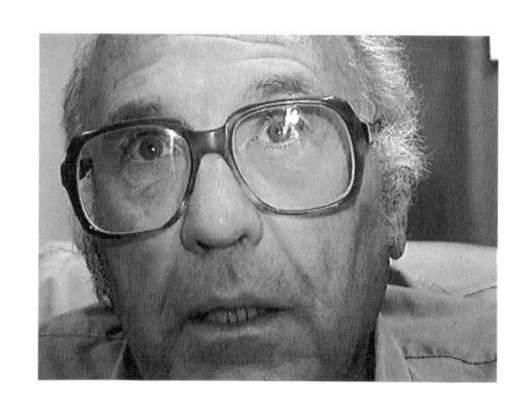

Psoriatic arthritis is one of the spondarthropathies which include Reiter's syndrome, ankylosing spondylitis and the arthritis of ulcerative colitis and Crohn's disease. It occurs in 5% of those with psoriasis, often involves two or three proximal joints of the hands or feet and generally has a better prognosis than rheumatoid arthritis. The exception is the rare patient, such as the one here, in whom a severe destructive form of psoriatic arthropathy, known as arthritis mutilans, occurs. In this condition, ankylosis of the joints, dissolution of bone (pencil and cup) and telescoping of the fingers occur. In many cases, the arthritis is similar to that seen in rheumatoid arthritis, as it is a synovitis that may involve almost any joint in the body. Unlike rheumatoid arthritis, it is usually asymmetrical and tends to involve the distal interphalangeal and sacroiliac joints. Over 80% of patients with psoriatic arthropathy have involvement of the nails, with thimble pitting, thickening, onycholysis (separation of the nail-plate from the nail-bed) and ridging.

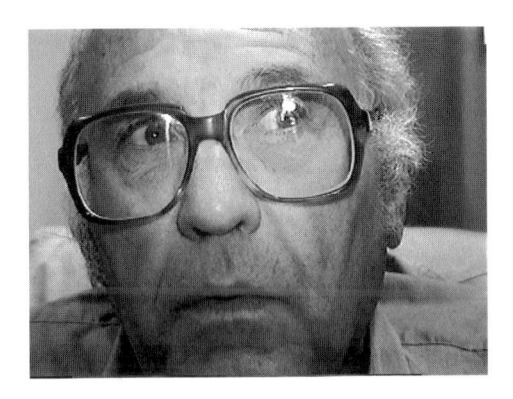

Basic science

Spondarthropathies

There is a very strong association between the inherited antigen HLA-B27 and ankylosing spondylitis. No fewer than 96% of patients with ankylosing spondylitis are HLA-B27 positive, compared with 7% of the general population. The risk of developing the disease in those born with the antigen is enhanced 300-fold. Even so, the chance of developing ankylosing spondylitis in those born HLA-B27 positive is only about 5% in men and 0.6% in women. The acute arthritis of Reiter's disease, which, in susceptible individuals, can follow sexually transmitted urethritis or *Shigella-*, *Salmonella-* or *Yersinia*-mediated dysentery, largely occurs in HLA-B27-positive individuals.

Patients with ulcerative colitis or Crohn's disease are 30 times more likely to develop spondylitis as the rest of the population. It is not a complication of inflammatory bowel disease as such, as in many patients it is evident for years before the bowel manifestations of the disease become manifest.

MCQs

1 The spondarthropathies usually present with pain and stiffness in the back.
2 Arthritis mutilans is the most typical arthritis associated with psoriasis.
3 Arthritis mutilans is characteristically exquisitely painful.
4 The chance of an HLA-B27-positive individual developing ankylosing spondylitis is 40%.
5 Patients with inflammatory bowel disease are predisposed to ankylosing spondarthropathies.

Case 46
The man with a sore foot

History

A 65-year-old motor engineer was seen by his GP with a painful right fifth toe. He was a keen walker and runner who, after one particular hike, had noticed that the outer border of his right fifth toe was sore and abraded. Despite attempts to heal it using various creams, dressings and changes in footwear, it became worse and, when the surrounding tissues turned dusky grey, his wife insisted that he 'get something done'. Previously, he had always been fit and well, and he was a lifelong non-smoker. There was no history of polyuria or polydipsia, and his only complaints on direct questioning were tiredness, which he had put down to ageing, blotchy hands, which seemed to worsen in cold weather, and a sense of fullness in the head with the sound of blood rushing in his ears, particularly at night. On examination, the tip of his spleen was palpable. His blood glucose level was $6.7\,mmol\,L^{-1}$. A full blood count showed a haemoglobin level of $15.1\,g\,dL^{-1}$, with a mean corpuscular volume (MCV) of $74\,fL$ (normal range = $80-96\,fL$), a white cell count of $18.6 \times 10^9\,L^{-1}$ (normal range = $4-11 \times 10^9\,L^{-1}$) and a platelet count of $998 \times 10^9\,L^{-1}$ (normal range = $150-400 \times 10^9\,L^{-1}$).

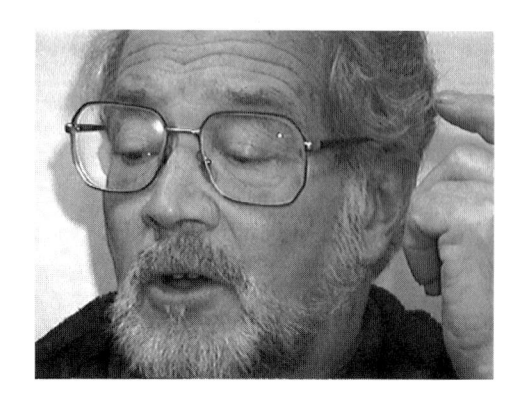

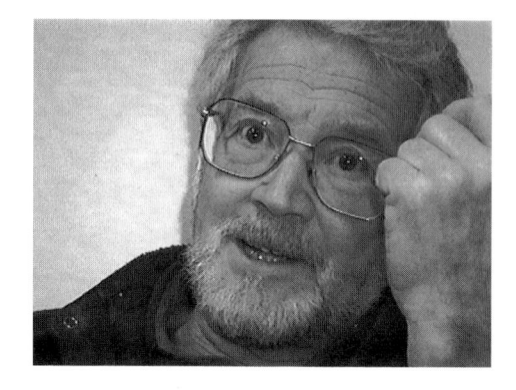

Notes

The patient had developed polycythaemia rubra vera.

The diagnosis of polycythaemia rubra vera was made on the basis of a modestly raised haemoglobin level despite iron deficiency (microcytosis) and the very high platelet count. Thrombocytosis is present in ≈50% of patients with polycythaemia rubra vera, but rarely rises to over $1000 \times 10^9\,L^{-1}$. Duodenal ulceration is also relatively common (affecting 8–10% of patients), and the tendency to bleed into the gastrointestinal tract in this condition was almost certainly responsible for the microcytic picture seen in this case. Leucocytosis is common in polycythaemia rubra vera, in keeping with the myeloproliferative nature of the condition, and a proportion of cases terminate in acute myeloid leukaemia or myelofibrosis as part of the natural history of the disease.

Thrombotic complications of polycythaemia rubra vera are common, and myocardial infarction, intermittent claudication and peripheral ischaemia (which led to the patient's foot problem) are typical. The elevated haematocrit is associated with itching, particularly after bathing, and a predisposition to gout. The increase in blood viscosity leads to symptoms such as dizziness, headaches, tinnitus, vertigo and rushing in the ears, thought to be related to disturbance of the cerebral circulation.

Polycythaemia rubra vera must be distinguished from secondary polycythaemia and relative polycythaemia.

- Secondary polycythaemia occurs physiologically in response to sustained hypoxia, such as that found in chronic obstructive pulmonary disease, alveolar hypoventilation, sustained high altitude and right to left shunts (e.g. cavernous haemangiomas of the lung and congenital cyanotic heart disease), and rarely in renal or hepatic tumours producing erythropoietins.
- Relative polycythaemia occurs when the red cell count is raised because of a reduction in plasma volume (associated with hypertension and vascular disease).

Basic science

Erythropoiesis

The earliest recognizable precursor of erythrocytes in the bone marrow is the proerythroblast. This gives rise to early, intermediate and late erythroblasts, characterized by increasing levels of mature haemoglobin, progressive loss of RNA coding for haemoglobin and, finally, loss of nucleoli and extrusion of the nuclear remnant to become a marrow reticulocyte. After 2 days, the marrow reticulocyte passes into the peripheral circulation and, after a further 24–48 h, loses the final remnants of blue-staining RNA and decreases slightly in size to become a mature erythrocyte. Under maximum stimulation, the bone marrow is capable of increasing its production of red cells by up to eightfold. Red cells are ≈7 μm in diameter under normal conditions and have a volume of 80–96 fL. Changes in red cell size are useful diagnostically.

Differential diagnosis of macrocytosis

- Megaloblastic anaemia:
    Folate deficiency: for example, dietary; coeliac disease; pregnancy; antifolate drugs.
    Vitamin B_{12} deficiency: for example, pernicious anaemia; Crohn's disease of the terminal ileum; dietary.
- Reticulocytosis:
    For example, following haemorrhage.
- Alcohol (chronic ingestion).
- Liver disease.
- Myelomatosis.
- Hypothyroidism.
- Acquired sideroblastic anaemia.
- Aplastic anaemia.
- Cytotoxic drugs (e.g. azathioprine).
- Anticonvulsants.

Differential diagnosis of microcytosis

- Iron deficiency:
    Blood loss: menorrhagia; gastrointestinal bleeding; haematuria.
    Dietary: especially vegetarians.
    Increased requirements: for example, pregnancy; infants and adolescents.
    Malabsorption: for example, coeliac disease; atrophic gastritis.
- Anaemia of chronic disease (normal iron stores).
- Thalassaemia trait.
- Sideroblastic anaemia:
    Primary.
    Secondary: alcoholism; lead poisoning; carcinoma; myeloproliferative disorders.
- Thyrotoxicosis.
- Giant platelet syndrome.

MCQs

1 Patients with polycythaemia rubra vera have an increased risk of developing leukaemia.

2 Myocardial infarction and peripheral ischaemia are typical complications of polycythaemia.
3 Microcytosis is associated with iron deficiency, thalassaemia trait and thyrotoxicosis.
4 Hyperviscosity is associated predominantly with gastrointestinal signs such as bleeding.
5 Secondary causes of polycythaemia include sustained hypoxia and left to right shunts.

Case 47
Recurrent gastrointestinal bleeding

History

An 85-year-old man was admitted with a long history of bleeding and anaemia, and a short history of vomiting 'coffee grounds'. His father suffered from recurrent bouts of uncontrolled bleeding throughout his life and eventually died in his fifties of uncontrolled rectal bleeding. The patient had known from the age of 12 years that he was predisposed to bleeding. Contact sports, such as rugby, would invariably be accompanied by bruising which was sometimes severe, and as a young man he bled continually for 2 weeks after having nine teeth extracted by a dentist. He had undergone several blood transfusions over the previous 20 years, but had been perfectly well on long-term iron supplements for several years until the bout of nausea on the morning of admission.

The four siblings of the patient were not troubled by the bleeding diathesis, but both the patient's daughter and one of his granddaughters were mildly affected.

Examination was entirely unremarkable. His platelet count was well within normal limits ($300\,000\,mm^{-3}$), but his bleeding time was moderately prolonged. In view of his history, an upper gastrointestinal endoscopy was not carried out.

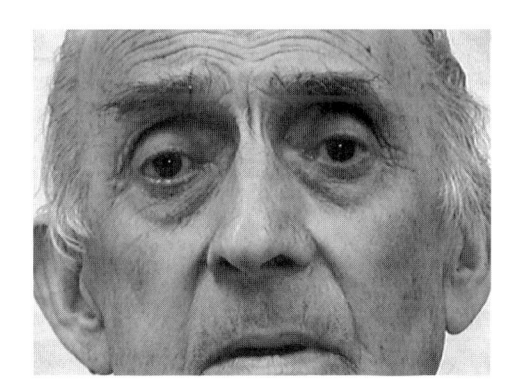

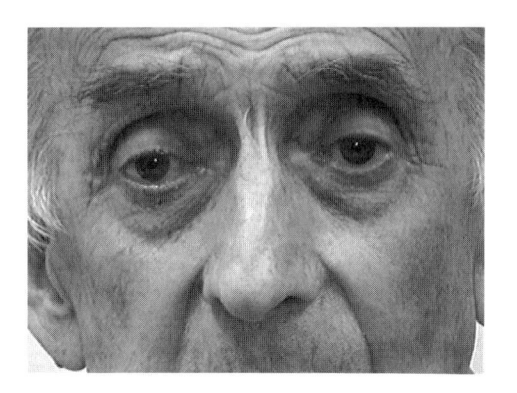

Notes

The patient had von Willebrand's disease.

von Willebrand's disease is an autosomal dominant condition with a prevalence of 0.1%, and is the most common inherited bleeding disorder. von Willebrand's factor is a complex plasma glycoprotein that acts as a carrier protein for factor VIII, and also facilitates platelet adhesion after vessel injury by forming a bridge between vascular sub-endothelium and platelet membrane receptors. A modest reduction in von Willebrand's factor is enough to cause bleeding, which usually occurs after trauma or surgery. In more severely affected cases, spontaneous genitourinary, gastrointestinal and nasopharyngeal bleeding are common. Because the glycoprotein is produced by the normal allele and is increased during systemic inflammation, pregnancy and central nervous system disorders, like other acute phase proteins, circulating levels of von Willebrand's factor may at times be relatively normal even in affected people.

The condition can be treated with cryoprecipitate, a blood product rich in von Willebrand's factor, with oral contraceptives, which moderate excessive menstrual blood loss, or with 1-desamino-8-D-arginine vasopressin (DDAVP), which raises the level of von Willebrand's factor.

Basic science

Clotting disorders due to platelet/vessel wall problems

Patients with platelet or vessel wall disorders tend to bleed immediately after trauma into superficial sites, such as the skin, mucous membranes or the gastrointestinal or genitourinary tracts. In contrast, patients with disorders of coagulation bleed into deep subcutaneous tissues, muscles, joints or body cavities hours or days later. Bleeding associated with the common disorders of platelet and vessel wall, such as von Willebrand's disease, drug-induced platelet dysfunction and the various causes of thrombocytopenia, tends to respond to simple, physical measures, such as pressure or packing, steroids or platelet or plasma factor transfusion. In contrast, the chronic, severe bleeding associated with coagulation disorders usually warrants more specialized and long-term medical therapy to prevent chronic disability or death.

The 'bleeding time' is a sensitive measure of platelet function. A bleeding time of over 10 min is associated with a moderate increase in the risk of bleeding. The risk of haemorrhage is high if bleeding time exceeds 15 or 20 min.

Patients with platelet counts of less than 50 000 mm^{-3} have an increased risk of bruising, and the development of purpura or bleeding from mucous membranes immediately after mild trauma. If the platelet count falls to less than 20 000 mm^{-3}, there is a risk of spontaneous bleeding which may occur internally or intracranially.

Causes of thrombocytopenia

- Decreased marrow production:
  Marrow infiltrated: tumour or fibrosis (myelofibrosis).
  Marrow failure: aplasia or hypoplasia.
- Splenic sequestration:
  Splenomegaly: tumour or portal hypertension.
- Increased platelet destruction:
  Non-immune: intravascular prosthesis, such as cardiac valves; disseminated intravascular coagulation; sepsis; vasculitis.
  Immune: autoantibodies to platelet antigens; drug-associated antibodies; circulating immune complexes, such as those found in systemic lupus erythematosus (SLE), bacteraemia or viraemia.

Platelet production

Platelets are small, granulated bodies between 2 and 4 µm in diameter. They are produced by the fragmentation of megakaryocytes, which are very large bone marrow cells that have undergone several cycles of DNA replication without cell division, making them strikingly polyploid. Around one-third of all platelets produced are sequestered by the spleen, but the remainder circulate for 7–10 days, become senescent and are removed from the circulation. Platelet numbers are maintained between about 150×10^9 and $400 \times 10^9 \, L^{-1}$, but can increase rapidly in systemic inflammation, tumours, haemorrhage and in mild iron deficiency anaemia (reactive thrombocytosis).

MCQs

1 von Willebrand's disease is the most common inherited bleeding disorder.
2 DDAVP reduces bleeding in von Willebrand's disease.

3 Patients with platelet disorders tend to bleed into muscles and joints rather than the skin.
4 In von Willebrand's disease, von Willebrand's factor levels are invariably low.
5 In portal hypertension, splenomegaly can lead to thrombocytopenia.

Case 48
Episodic palpitations

History

A 27-year-old woman was seen in the outpatient department with a long history of intermittent palpitations. They occurred about once every week on average, and could come on at any time. Each time, the onset as well as the resolution of the very fast, regular palpitations would be abrupt and would, in most cases, be accompanied by a feeling of faintness. On a few occasions, the patient had passed out during the attacks, but mostly she remained conscious. For several minutes after the end of each attack, apart from feeling relief, she also felt very tired, but had not noticed a particular urge to pass water. There was no history of sweating, flushing, abdominal discomfort or headaches related to the attacks, and the palpitations were invariably rapid and regular. Between attacks she felt completely well, although, as the attacks had become more frequent, her general level of anxiety had increased. She had no significant past medical history and did not smoke. An ECG between attacks of palpitations was diagnostic.

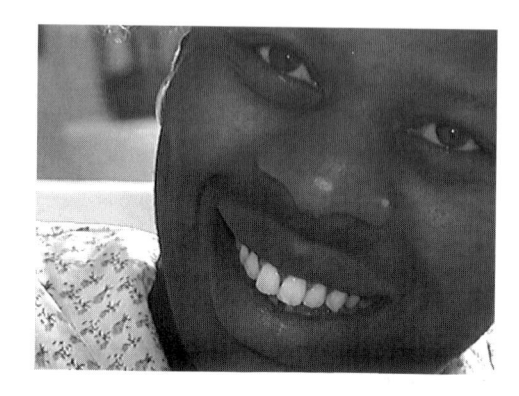

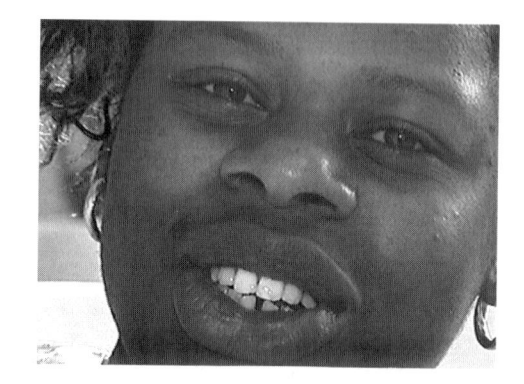

Notes

The patient had Wolff–Parkinson–White syndrome with a left-sided aberrant conducting pathway.

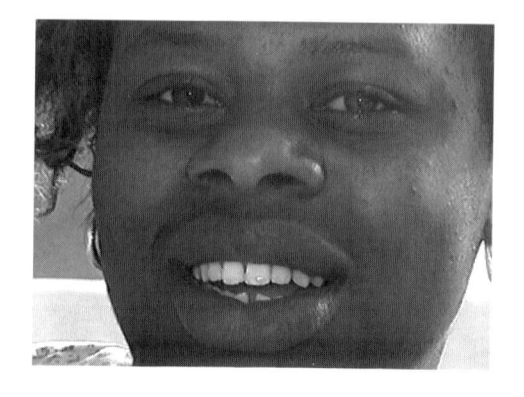

Four different types of pre-excitation are caused by conducting strands of muscle fibres bridging the insulating valve rings that, under normal circumstances, provide effective electrical insulation between the atria and the ventricles. The likely position of the abnormal bundle can be determined approximately from the pattern of the 12-lead ECG. R waves in V1 and V2 indicate a left-sided aberrant conducting pathway and Q waves in the same chest leads indicate a right-sided aberrant conducting pathway. A positive QRS complex in the inferior leads (II, III and aVF) indicates a lateral bundle, and a predominantly negative QRS complex in the inferior leads indicates a septal bundle.

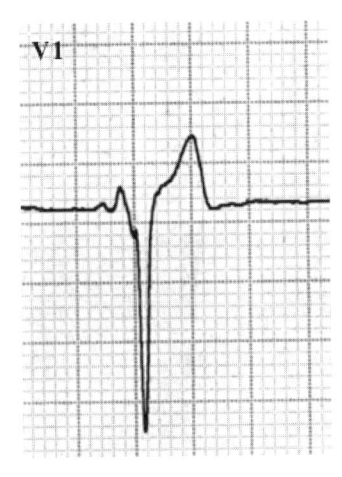

Once localized, the short circuiting muscle bundle can be ablated with radiofrequency current applied from the endocardium during catheter studies to effect a cure.

One of the most important features in her history was that the palpitations ended abruptly. There are many causes of palpitations, and many symptoms that patients tend to refer to as palpitations. The rapidity of the onset of palpitations is a non-specific symptom as patients almost invariably become aware of their presence abruptly. The pattern of resolution of palpitations, however, is much more informative, as those resulting from anxiety tend to resolve slowly, whereas those mediated by aberrant conduction, whatever the cause, are either there or not there. Intuitively, it is clear that an abrupt resolution of the dysrhythmia is almost invariable *in a conduction defect* and that a gradual resolution of palpitations (as is more often the case in anxiety attacks or catecholamine release from a phaeochromocytoma) militates against the presence of a conduction defect as the cause.

Basic science

Cardiac cell depolarization

With the exception of cells of the sinoatrial and atrioventricular nodes, the interior of cardiac cells in the resting state is maintained at a negative potential of 80–90 mV, almost entirely due to an electrochemical potassium ion gradient across their membranes. The activation of cardiac cells is affected by transient depolarization (an action potential), the ionic nature of which depends, to some extent, on the location of the cells being examined. Most of the initial depolarization is caused by rapid sodium influx into myocardial cells, followed by a somewhat slower influx of calcium ions. In myocardial cells that exhibit automaticity, the resting potential decreases spontaneously towards the threshold potential at which a full depolarizing ion flux occurs.

After depolarization, myocardial cells are absolutely refractory (to a stimulus of any strength) for a time and then become relatively refractory for a further period (during which a stimulus cannot elicit a full, propagated response) before returning to full excitability.

The sinoatrial node, at the junction of the right atrium and superior vena cava, is the normal cardiac pacemaker because it has the fastest intrinsic discharge rate. It is responsible for the increase in heart rate (tachycardia) that occurs with sympathetic stimulation and the decrease in heart rate during sleep. Dysfunction of the sinoatrial node, usually presumed to be ischaemic in origin in the elderly, produces episodes of bradycardia and tachycardia.

MCQs

1 Wolff–Parkinson–White syndrome can be cured.
2 In Wolff–Parkinson–White syndrome, R waves in V1 and V2 indicate a left-sided aberrant conducting pathway.
3 Dysrhythmias due to

Wolff–Parkinson–White syndrome are usually perceived as abrupt in onset and remission.
4 The negative potential of myocardial cells is predominantly due to a sodium ion gradient.
5 In sinoatrial node cells, the resting potential increases spontaneously towards the threshold.

Case 49
Refractory hypertension

History

A 73-year-old retired post office engineer was admitted to hospital for the investigation of persistent hypertension. He had spent over 4 years in hospital as a child following an episode of rheumatic fever, and subsequently became a postman and successful amateur sportsman. As far as he was concerned, apart from the episode of severe illness as a child, he had been perfectly well throughout his life. He had suffered from a raised blood pressure for as long as he could remember. The hypertension was untreated and, as far as he was concerned, it was 'normal for him'.

On examination, the findings of note were a blood pressure of 194/110 mmHg (in both arms) with a regular pulse of 80 beats per minute. The apex beat was displaced into the anterior axillary line and, although heart sounds were normal, a bruit was heart on auscultation of his chest wall bilaterally at the back. Palpation of his peripheral pulses revealed marked brachiofemoral delay, but was otherwise unremarkable. Fundoscopy showed mild hypertensive retinopathy only.

An ECG was normal. The diagnosis was made from the chest X-ray, which showed a normal-sized heart and normal lung fields.

Notes

The patient had coarctation of the aorta.

In addition to the normal-sized heart and normal lung fields, the chest X-ray revealed

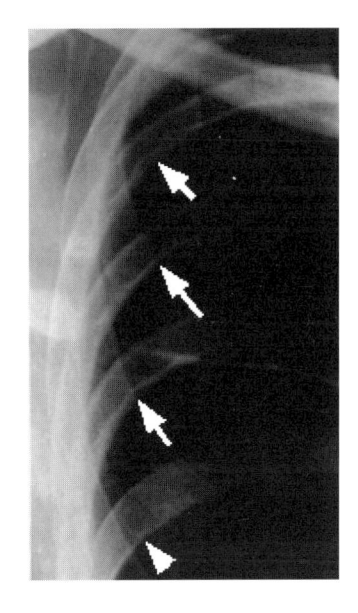

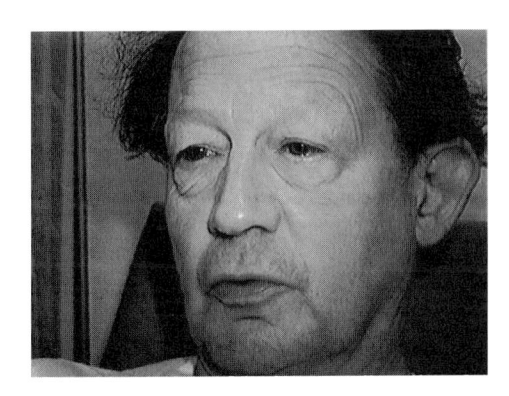

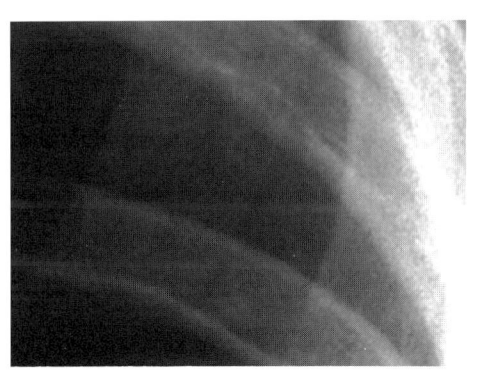

Normal pattern   Preductal   Postductal

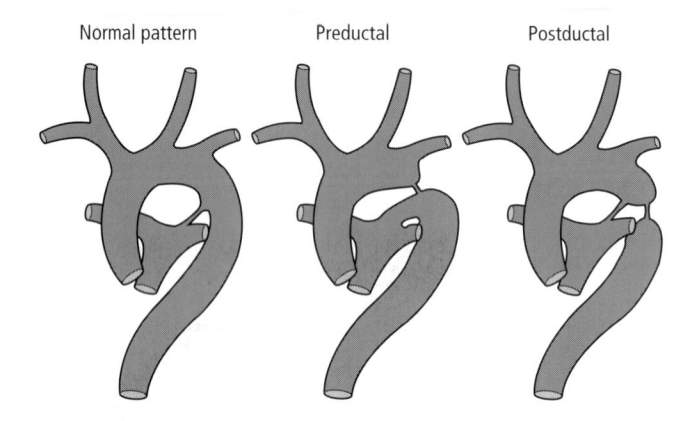

bilateral notching of the inferior border of the ribs posteriorly.

In coarctation of the aorta, the aortic lumen above, or more usually below, the junction of the ductus arteriosus (below the origin of the left subclavian artery) is narrowed. When the narrowing is above the ductus arteriosus, the latter usually remains patent in postnatal life. When the narrowing is below the ductus arteriosus, the ductus arteriosus involutes as normal and the intercostal and internal thoracic arteries dilate to form a satisfactory collateral circulation. This is often audible as a bruit on direct auscultation over the vessels, and the chronic pulsatile pressure exerted on adjacent structures leads to bone remodelling that produces the characteristic rib notching.

Coarctation occurs in 7% of patients with congenital heart disease, and is more common in males than females. Associated cardiac anomalies include valvular defects, such as bicuspid or stenosed aortic valve or mitral regurgitation, and ventricular septal defects. Most patients, as is the case here, are asymptomatic, but headache, epistaxis and claudication with exercise can occur depending on the severity of stenosis. Treatment is surgical.

Basic science

Development of the aortic arch

The first major blood vessels to develop in the early embryo are the paired dorsal aortas. These loop backwards in the first pharyngeal arch, either side of the pharyngeal gut, then run along the axis of the 3-week-old embryo from the developing heart. As each subsequent pharyngeal arch develops, a new pair (neoaortic arch) of arteries is formed. All six pairs of pharyngeal arches and their corresponding arteries are not present simultaneously. Their involution, by the time the embryo is 14 mm long, leaves a left-sided aortic arch (between the left common carotid and the left subclavian arteries) formed from the fourth arch, fed from the right ventricle via the ductus arteriosus, a distal portion of the sixth aortic arch.

MCQs

1. Coarctation of the aorta is associated with a patent ductus arteriosus.
2. *In utero*, the left-sided aortic arch is fed from the left ventricle via the ductus arteriosus.
3. Marfan's syndrome and Turner's syndrome are associated with coarctation of the aorta.
4. Most patients with coarctation of the aorta are asymptomatic.
5. A murmur heard over the upper back is typical of aortic coarctation.

Case 50
Cyanosis and breathlessness

History

A 19-year-old university student was seen in clinic with a number of problems, the most prominent of which were long-standing breathlessness and paroxysmal ventricular tachycardias. She had been born with an almost complete atrioventricular septal defect and multiple ventricular septal defects. Pulmonary hypertension developed in childhood, and her exercise tolerance, which had always been much less than her peers, diminished further with time. The only effective medication for her ventricular dysrhythmias was found to be amiodarone, and this unfortunately induced thyroiditis, the effects of which further exacerbated her breathlessness. Despite surgery in childhood, a substantial ventricular septal defect remained and, over the years, the patient had become increasingly cyanosed.

Notes

The patient had Eisenmenger's syndrome.

The patient was born with a ventricular septal defect which allowed extensive shunting throughout her life. Initially left to right, as pulmonary pressure inexorably increased, the shunt stopped and eventually reversed (Eisenmenger's syndrome). Once right to left shunting starts, deoxygenated blood enters the systemic circulation and central and peripheral cyanosis becomes pronounced. Under these circumstances, attempts to close the defect between the left and right sides of the circulation invariably provide little symptomatic relief at best and often result in mortality.

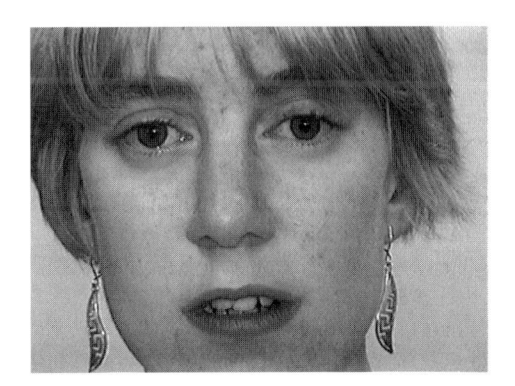

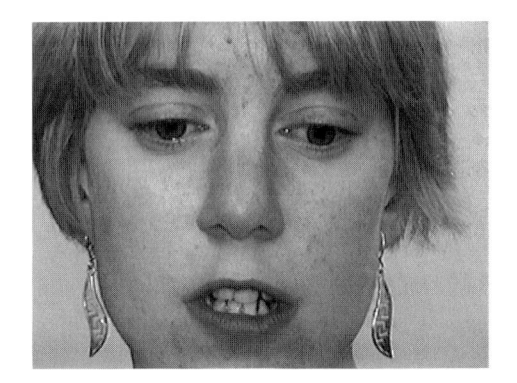

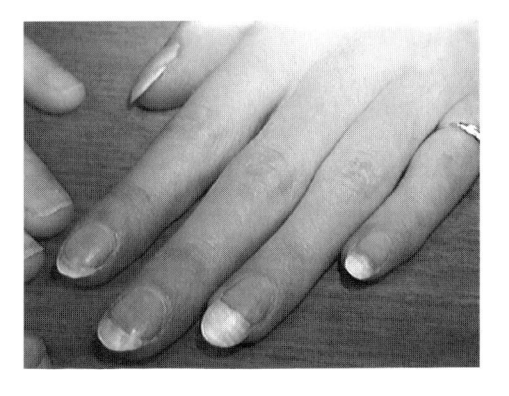

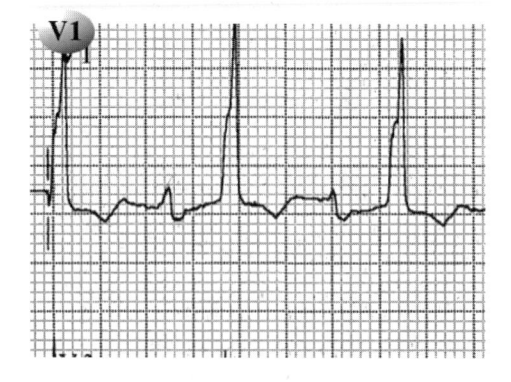

Secondary pulmonary hypertension

Pulmonary hypertension (a pulmonary artery pressure of 20 mmHg or greater at rest and at least 30 mmHg on exercise with a normal pulmonary artery occlusion pressure) is a common accompaniment to many cardiorespiratory disorders. The causes of increased pulmonary resistance are complex, and include increased pulmonary blood flow and blood pressure, hypoxia, acidosis and polycythaemia. Cyanotic congenital heart disease is a particular risk factor, as is a large ventricular septal defect. Under normal circumstances, dilatation of the pulmonary vascular bed prevents any significant increase in pulmonary pressure unless pulmonary flow is greatly increased. The increase in pulmonary pressure in congenital heart disease is often the result of increased pulmonary resistance at the level of the pulmonary arterioles.

Basic science

Embryology of the heart

Longitudinal growth of the heart tube during the first month of embryonic life is accompanied by complex folding and the development of septa which divide the fetal heart into chambers.

Atrial septum formation. The communication between the primitive atria, the ostium primum, gradually closes as the septum primum grows. As it does so, part of its upper wall breaks down to form the ostium secundum, which maintains a communication between the atria. The direction of flow, right to left, is enforced by the rigidity of a second leaf of tissue, the septum secundum, which grows down to overlap the ostium secundum on the right side, leaving the septum primum to act as a flap valve. This right to left shunt, bypassing the right ventricle and pulmonary circulation, is closed at birth by a number of factors, including the dramatic fall in pulmonary resistance that follows the newborn's first breath.

Interventricular septum formation. The communication between the primitive ventricles is closed largely by rapid growth of ventricular muscle and fusion of the medial walls of the left and right ventricles to form the muscular interventricular septum. Above the top of the septum, a pair of obliquely placed 'truncus swellings' fuse to form the spiral aorticopulmonary septum that separates the pulmonary and aortic channels. This process, together with further outgrowths of tissue from the top of the muscular interventricular septum, completes the division of the ventricles into left and right.

Atrial septum abnormalities. In about 20% of adults, the septum secundum and septum primum do not completely fuse, and it is possible to pass a probe from the right to the left atrium. Defects in or absence of the septum secundum results in an 'atrial septal defect' which can lead to a number of problems in adult life. The complete absence of the atrial septum is most serious and, as in this patient, is always associated with other serious defects elsewhere in the heart.

Interventricular septum abnormalities. The formation of the upper, membranous part of the interventricular septum is complex, and it is not surprising that small defects are relatively frequent.

The most common abnormality of the truncus and conus—the pads of tissue that separate the pulmonary and aortic channels and complete the upper, membranous part of the interventricular septum—is tetralogy of Fallot. In this condition, uneven division of the conus results in narrowing of the right ventricular outflow region, leading to pulmonary stenosis and right ventricular hypertrophy, and a medially displaced aorta above a high ventricular septal defect.

Failure of the truncus to divide results in 'persistent truncus arteriosus', in which the pulmonary artery arises a little way up a common vessel that becomes the aorta. A truncoconal septum that fails to follow its normal spiral course, but is nevertheless complete, results in the aorta originating from the apex of the right ventricle, and the pulmonary artery arising from the left, so-called transposition of the great vessels.

MCQs

1 The septum secundum overlaps the ostium secundum on the left side.
2 In 20% of adults, the septum secundum and septum primum do not fuse completely.
3 Ventricular septal defect is one of the components of tetralogy of Fallot.
4 Developmental defects of the truncoconal septum result in atrial septal defects.
5 Chronic obstructive pulmonary disease is associated with pulmonary hypertension.

MCQ answers

Case 1

1 **False** Toxoplasma encephalitis, caused by the ubiquitous intracellular protozoan *Toxoplasma gondii*, is the most common focal central nervous system infection complicating acquired immunodeficiency syndrome (AIDS).
2 **False** The domestic cat is the only host of intraintestinal *Toxoplasma* oocytes, and therefore the primary route of human infection is ingestion of food contaminated with cat droppings.
3 **True** Remarkably, the new protease inhibitor combination drug therapies appear to be able to achieve this in some individuals, including the patient illustrated here.
4 **False** It is a RNA retrovirus, classified as a lentivirus. Its genome is coded as RNA, but reverse transcribed to DNA before integration into the host's genome.
5 **False** The principal target of human immunodeficiency virus (HIV) is the CD4+ T-helper cell because of the affinity of a glycoprotein component of the viral envelope (gp120) with the CD4 molecule.

Case 2

1 **False** Only 10% of cases are associated with malignancy.
2 **True** The purplish rash over the metacarpophalangeal joints is characteristic. In children, oedema of the eyelids is associated with a characteristic heliotrope discoloration.
3 **True** The 'bulb' refers to the medulla oblongata. Bulbar palsy is lower motor neurone paralysis affecting the glossopharyngeal, vagus and hypoglossal nerves. Pseudobulbar palsy is upper motor neurone paralysis of the same. Like any other upper motor neurone lesion, increased tone is characteristic.
4 **True** Muscle enzymes are raised.
5 **False** Around one-third of patients have residual muscle weakness, and fibrous tissue within muscles can lead to contractures.

Case 3

1 **False** Decussation of the corticospinal tracts occurs in the medulla. Below that level, damage to these tracts produces ipsilateral effects.
2 **False** Fine touch, vibration and proprioception are mediated by the posterior columns which decussate in the brain stem. Unlike spinothalamic damage, the effects are ipsilateral.
3 **True** The mid-thoracic spine and the sacroiliac joints are typical sites of tuberculous involvement.
4 **False** The incidence of tuberculous osteomyelitis is only 1–3%.
5 **True** Acute intervertebral disc herniation and vertebral collapse due to neoplastic infiltration account for most of these cases.

Case 4

1 **False** As disconnection of the vagus nerve doubles the resting heart rate, parasympathetic tone predominates.
2 **True** The vasomotor centre is located in the medulla oblongata.
3 **True** Sinus dysrhythmia, the fluctuation in pulse rate and pressure during respiration,

normally results in tachycardia with reduced pulse volume on inspiration and bradycardia with an increase in pulse pressure on expiration.
4 **True** It receives afferents from cardiac and arterial baroreceptors.
5 **True** These block parasympathetic activity and lead to tachycardia.

Case 5

1 **False** The prevalence is about right, but the condition is dominantly inherited.
2 **True** The skeletal deformities give rise to the 'Marfanoid habitus'. Structural abnormalities of the great vessels predispose them to aneurysmal dilatation and dissection; the weakness of the suspensory ligaments of the lens allows it to dislocate, usually upwards.
3 **False** New mutations account for only 15–30% of cases.
4 **False** They are usually painless.
5 **True** Kaposi's sarcoma is commonly associated with human immunodeficiency virus (HIV) infection.

Case 6

1 **False** The process is generally thought to be mediated by immune complex deposition.
2 **False** This pattern is typical of Wegener's granulomatosis. In polyarteritis nodosa, renal and visceral rather than pulmonary vessels are usually involved.
3 **False** Antineutrophil cytoplasmic antibodies (ANCAs) are positive in 90% of cases. Unfortunately, the specificity of a positive ANCA is poor.
4 **True** The reason for the association of polyarteritis nodosa and hepatitis B positivity is unclear, but the two are strongly associated.
5 **True** Almost all patients with Churg–Strauss disease have a history of asthma. Systemic vasculitis involving at least two extrapulmonary organs is required to make the diagnosis.

Case 7

1 **True** Early menarche, late menopause and exposure to exogenous oestrogens all increase the risk of breast cancer.
2 **False** Small, oestrogen receptor-expressing tumours without axillary nodal involvement in a postmenopausal woman are associated with the most favourable prognosis.
3 **False** Human chorionic gonadotrophin is a marker of trophoblastic and gonadal tumours. Carcinoembryonic antigen is a marker of cancers of the colon, pancreas, stomach, lung and breast.
4 **True** Levels are raised in 70% of patients with hepatocellular carcinoma, testicular teratomas and, occasionally, with gastrointestinal tumours.
5 **False** Most cases of hypercalcaemia in malignancy are due to the production of parathyroid hormone-related peptide or other calcaemic factors by the tumour rather than by bone involvement. The exception is breast cancer, where hypercalcaemia is usually associated with bone metastases.

Case 8

1 **False** Neurofibromatosis is the most common of this group of diseases (the phakomatoses) with an incidence approaching 1 : 3000 per annum.
2 **True** *Café-au-lait* patches are the most common skin features of neurofibromatosis. Typically, more than five are present, each greater than 2.5 cm in diameter.
3 **True** Gliomas, acoustic neuromas, meningiomas and phaeochromocytomas (which can occur intracranially) are all more prevalent.
4 **False** The cephalic and caudal ends of the

neural tube are closed within the first month of the first trimester.
5 **True** The midbrain is formed from the mesencephalon, and the pons, cerebellum and medulla oblongata are derived from the rhombencephalon.

Case 9

1 **True** The incidence of phaeochromocytoma at unselected autopsy is ≈0.1%. Almost all of these are occult and, even when analysed in retrospect, fewer than 50% of such patients had a history of hypertension *in vivo*.
2 **False** Phaeochromocytomas are usually single and benign in adults. In children, they are more frequently bilateral, extra-adrenal and malignant.
3 **False** It is part of the multiple endocrine neoplasia 2a and 2b (MEN2a and MEN2b) syndromes. The MEN1 syndrome consists of tumours of the pituitary, parathyroids and pancreas.
4 **False** Although patients with phaeochromocytoma and paroxysmal symptoms can be very anxious, they are usually well between attacks. Patients with neuropsychiatric symptoms, in contrast, have attacks that last for hours or days rather than minutes to hours and are often 'ill' between attacks.
5 **False** They can occur in many tissues, including the eye, central nervous system and bone.

Case 10

1 **True** Around 1–3% of the adult population is affected, and most cases are diagnosed incidentally as a result of investigations for a raised alkaline phosphatase level or after an X-ray examination for other indications.
2 **False** The solid calcium and phosphate mineral phase (hydroxyapatite) of bone is deposited in close relationship to an organic matrix of mostly type I collagen and proteins, such as osteocalcin and osteonectin.
3 **False** The formation of the skull bones is by ossification within membranes rather than by ossification of the shaft and epiphyses of a cartilage template. Epiphyseal fusion stops the growth of long bones at the end of puberty.
4 **False** The *c-src* gene appears to be a critical regulator of osteoclast function, as its absence leads to osteopetrosis (marble bones rather than porotic bones).
5 **False** Even in extensive disease, which is quite rare in itself, the risk of osteosarcoma is only around 1%.

Case 11

1 **False** It is synthesized in the hypothalamus. The formation of a neoneurohypophysis after pituitary surgery means that postoperative diabetes insipidus has a reasonable chance of resolving of its own accord with time.
2 **True** In the latter, the patient is woken up at intervals throughout the night to pass water. In psychogenic polydipsia, the water load consumed before bedtime is often cleared within a few hours of retiring to bed and the latter half of the night is often undisturbed.
3 **False** A water deprivation test is not often required. The circumstances and symptoms are usually diagnostic.
4 **True** The aetiology of histiocytosis X is unknown, but 90% of patients are either current or former cigarette smokers.
5 **True** Many patients with the condition are between the ages of 20 and 40 years, and have one or two of these features.

Case 12

1 **False** The metabolic defect affects haem synthesis rather than catabolism. Haem catabolism leads to the formation of

non cyclic tetrapyrroles known as bile pigments.
2 **False** Porphobilinogen is excreted in the urine and, as it spontaneously polymerizes to produce pigmented products, the urine darkens on standing.
3 **False** At least two-thirds of those who inherit the condition do not develop clinical evidence of abnormal haem biosynthesis.
4 **True** The abdominal pain is often accompanied by vomiting, constipation, fever and a raised white cell count.
5 **False** As preformed porphyrins do not accumulate in the blood, a photosensitive rash does not occur in this type of porphyria.

Case 13

1 **True** Immunoglobulin A (IgA) nephropathy is the most common pattern of glomerulonephritis seen in areas of the world where renal biopsies are used in the diagnosis of renal failure.
2 **False** The deposits of IgA in IgA nephropathy are in the mesangium.
3 **True** End-stage renal failure is reached in 25% of patients 25 years after the diagnosis.
4 **True** The tubule also secretes substances into the filtrate.
5 **False** Molecules such as thyroxine and testosterone that are bound to plasma proteins largely escape filtration.

Case 14

1 **True** This distinguishes chronic renal failure from renal tubular acidosis, where sulphate and phosphate ions are excreted normally.
2 **False** In renal tubular acidosis, the kidneys are unable to excrete hydrogen ions. Potassium levels increase as hydrogen ions displace potassium ions out of cells.
3 **False** Metabolic acidosis is caused by the ingestion of non-volatile acids, decreased acid excretion by the kidneys or increased loss of alkali.
4 **False** In metabolic acidosis due to renal tubular acidosis or loss of alkali in diarrhoea, the anion gap is normal as plasma chloride is increased as much as bicarbonate is decreased.
5 **True** The normal range is 8–16 mmol L^{-1}, mostly due to the negative charge of plasma proteins, such as albumin, and, to a lesser extent, phosphate, sulphate and organic acid anions.

Case 15

1 **True** This test is used to confirm the presence of normal parathyroid hormone (PTH) receptors.
2 **True** In addition to the intrinsic hydrolytic activity of the α subunit itself, adenylyl cyclase, with which the guanosine triphosphate (GTP)-bound α subunit associates, and GTPase-activating peptides within the cell promote GTP hydrolysis to guanosine diphosphate (GDP) and allow the α subunit to reassociate with the βγ subunits.
3 **False** This scenario would suggest hypoparathyroidism rather than pseudohypoparathyroidism, where PTH levels are high, but the peptide is ineffective.
4 **True** Other skeletal manifestations, such as shortening of the metacarpals and metatarsals and short stature, are also evident.
5 **True** X-linked inheritance is characteristic.

Case 16

1 **False** Its point of origin is the foramen caecum, an indentation in the floor of the pharyngeal gut that becomes the intersection between the anterior two-thirds and the posterior third of the tongue.
2 **False** The incidence of congenital hypothyroidism is 1 : 4000–5000 births. Its

high incidence and serious long-term consequences make neonatal screening with a heal prick blood sample worthwhile.
3 **True** Many manifestations of the condition may be extremely subtle. Falling off the height centiles while tracking along the weight centiles is typical.
4 **True** Also, the amount present in meat depends on the amount in the animals' diets.
5 **False** It is a feature of hyperthyroidism and psoriasis.

Case 17

1 **True** Graves' eye disease can occur before thyroid disease and even entirely on its own. It can also be unilateral.
2 **True** In lagophthalmos, the forward movement of the globe of the eye is such that the lids fail to cover it fully when closed, or tend to drift apart during the night. This can lead to exposure keratitis.
3 **False** It is a sign of sympathetic overactivity which is a feature of all types of thyrotoxicosis.
4 **False** The mechanisms responsible are supranuclear, i.e. central to the cranial nerve nuclei.
5 **True** As the weak eye is least able to move towards the target, the image hits the retina away from the macula and is perceived as peripheral to the image cast by the normal eye.

Case 18

1 **True** Ultimately, these features occur in almost all patients with the condition.
2 **False** Hypotension, particularly postural hypotension, is found.
3 **False** Destruction of the adrenals abolishes aldosterone production causing hyponatraemia and hyperkalaemia, but biochemical changes are late and suggest impending Addisonian crisis.
4 **True** The normal response to stress is to increase circulating cortisol levels. Patients with Addison's disease cannot do this.
5 **True** Other autoimmune diseases, such as insulin-dependent diabetes, vitiligo, Hashimoto's disease and hypoparathyroidism, occur more commonly in patients with Addison's disease.

Case 19

1 **True** The condition may be obvious at birth or may become evident after an infection, such as chicken pox or infectious mononucleosis.
2 **True** There is a strong association with a series of metabolic disorders, including insulin resistance and hypertriglyceridaemia.
3 **False** Symptomatic coronary artery disease is rare.
4 **False** Lipodystrophy is one of the rare hypermetabolic syndromes in which relatively large numbers of calories can be ingested without weight gain.
5 **False** Hypertriglyceridaemia rather than hypercholesterolaemia is typical.

Case 20

1 **False** Prolactin is produced by anterior pituitary lactotroph (or mammotroph) cells only.
2 **False** Galactorrhoea in men is very unusual as it depends not just on prolactin, but on previous oestrogen priming of the breast.
3 **True** This very high level far exceeds the levels that would be expected in a microprolactinoma, during lactation or in response to pituitary stalk compression or stress.
4 **True** Unlike oxytocin levels, they do not rise in anticipation of suckling.
5 **False** Pituitary tumours can cause almost any kind of field loss. Unilateral changes are not at all unusual.

Case 21

1. **True** In pituitary disease, the thyroid continues to function, although at a reduced level. In primary hypothyroidism, the hypothyroidism is usually more profound.
2. **True** Self-reactive clones are deleted through mechanisms that are not clearly understood.
3. **True** The combination of hypothyroidism, hypoadrenalism and hypogonadism leads to this appearance.
4. **False** In the presence of low levels of circulating thyroid hormones, a thyroid-stimulating hormone (TSH) level within the 'normal range' is still inappropriately low. The same principle applies to the gonadotrophins.
5. **False** This function is carried out by T-lymphocyte, cell-mediated immunity. Activated B lymphocytes, in contrast, differentiate into plasma cells and produce antibodies that have particular affinities for foreign antigens that are free in the bloodstream or in other body fluids.

Case 22

1. **True** The presence of high levels of C peptide is a useful feature to distinguish endogenous from exogenous insulin excess.
2. **False** Insulinomas are rare tumours. Symptoms relieved by eating are common.
3. **False** About 50% of pancreatic insulin output is inactivated by the liver in first pass metabolism.
4. **True** Hypoglycaemic coma, caused by an accidental overdose of exogenous insulin, is rapidly reversed by an intramuscular injection of 1 mg glucagon. The patient can then be encouraged to take oral glucose.
5. **False** This would not be characteristic as many patients find that eating brings about symptomatic relief.

Case 23

1. **True** At least 10% of patients are mosaics.
2. **True** Routine karyotype analysis on peripheral white blood cells may miss the diagnosis in rare cases.
3. **False** There is no increased risk of testicular cancer. These patients do, however, have a modestly increased risk of breast cancer.
4. **False** The patients have primary hypogonadism, and follicle-stimulating hormone (FSH) and luteinizing hormone (LH) levels are usually raised.
5. **False** The first of the two cell divisions that constitute meiosis is preceded by chromosomal duplication.

Case 24

1. **True** In the extremely rare scenario of a pituitary adenoma in childhood producing excess growth hormone and causing hypogonadotrophic hypogonadism through compression of the normal pituitary, the lack of sex hormones leaves the epiphyses of long bones open and allows continued growth to occur.
2. **True** Growth during this time is extremely rapid.
3. **True** This allows for a more prolonged period of prepubertal growth which, together with a bigger growth spurt, accounts for the greater mean adult height in men.
4. **False** Growth hormone is responsible for limb growth, but growth of the axial skeleton is sex hormone mediated.
5. **True** In most cases, catch-up growth in small babies and 'catch-down' growth in large babies have occurred by this time, and individuals tend to track along the centiles.

Case 25

1. **False** Although thinning of the skin is induced by hypercortisolaemia, in

adrenocorticotrophic hormone (ACTH)-dependent disease, stimulation of adrenal pre-androgen production protects the skin against steroid-induced changes.
2 **False** Only 1% of cortisol is excreted in the urine unchanged. Most undergoes hepatic metabolism by reduction, oxidation, hydroxylation and conjugation reactions.
3 **False** The term refers to a group of enzyme defects in which the production of cortisol ± mineralocorticoids is defective, and ACTH drive to the adrenals is markedly increased in response.
4 **True** Individuals who are obese are usually strong, as merely carrying their weight around is a form of weight training. Proximal myopathy is a very characteristic finding in Cushing's syndrome.
5 **True** This steroid precursor is an important branch point of cortisol and preandrogen metabolism. As it is proximal to most enzyme defects responsible for congenital adrenal hyperplasia, it is characteristically elevated in the condition.

Case 26

1 **True** The chief source, however, is the choroid plexus.
2 **True** Such tenuous support for such a large organ is only possible because the density of the brain is only marginally more than that of the cerebrospinal fluid (CSF) that surrounds it. Although the mass of the brain is 1.4 kg, its submerged weight is only 50 g.
3 **False** The protein content of CSF is 0.3% of that of plasma, glucose levels are 65% of normal plasma levels, uric acid levels are one-third of plasma levels and lipids are virtually excluded from the CSF.
4 **False** Exclusion does not appear to be absolute. The blood–brain barrier is selective.
5 **True** The turnover of CSF is relatively rapid.

Case 27

1 **False** 5-Hydroxyindoleacetic acid is the urinary marker of excessive 5-hydroxytryptamine (5-HT) production.
2 **True** This is the classical triad of flushing, produced by episodic high levels of 5-HT, a right heart murmur due to endomyocardial fibrosis distorting the tricuspid valve and hepatomegaly (and sometimes the primary tumour) causing an abdominal mass.
3 **True** This is the classical triad of symptoms.
4 **False** Patients can live for many years despite the presence of hepatic metastases at diagnosis.
5 **True** The B vitamins nicotinic acid (niacin) and riboflavin are used to make the important coenzymes nicotinamide adenine dinucleotide (NAD) and flavin adenine dinucleotide (FAD), respectively.

Case 28

1 **True** A family history of recurrent gastrointestinal and nasal bleeding is typical of the condition.
2 **False** Vessel wall disorders are characterized by mild but recurrent bleeding from the skin and mucous membranes.
3 **True** Streptococcal pharyngitis is often the predisposing infection.
4 **False** Disseminated intravascular coagulation is not a feature of the condition.
5 **False** They are widespread, occurring, for example, in the liver and skin, but are often most troublesome in the gastrointestinal tract, nasal airways and lung.

Case 29

1 **False** Primary biliary cirrhosis is a diffuse, non-suppurative cholangitis that progressively destroys medium and small

bile ducts over a period of months to several years.
2 **True** The first clinical sign of primary biliary cirrhosis is usually persistent, generalized itching, followed by the development of dark urine, pale stools and jaundice.
3 **False** Once in the gall-bladder, a large portion of the salts is reabsorbed from hepatic bile leaving an aqueous solution containing cholesterol that is kept in solution by bile acids.
4 **True** The bile acid pool (of about 4 g) is circulated several times a day, with faecal losses of about 0.5 g daily.
5 **False** Gallstones develop in one in three women and one in five men, and at least two-thirds of each remain asymptomatic.

Case 30

1 **False** Serum copper levels are low.
2 **True** If a careful slit lamp examination fails to show these brown, gold or green corneal rings, the diagnosis of Wilson's disease is excluded.
3 **False** They are rare before this age.
4 **True** Excess hepatic copper levels prevent the formation of ceruloplasmin from apoceruloplasmin and copper. About 5% of patients with Wilson's disease have normal ceruloplasmin levels.
5 **False** Penicillamine needs to be continued lifelong and without interruption.

Case 31

1 **True** Conversely, about 30% of patients who develop epilepsy between the ages of 30 and 50 years harbour brain tumours.
2 **False** Metastases from extracranial neoplasms account for 23% of intracranial tumours.
3 **False** The symptoms of frontal lobe tumours are often subtle, and they frequently attain a considerable size before the patient presents.

4 **False** They account for about 20% of the total.
5 **False** Although slow growth can be accommodated by the brain, masses more than 3 cm in diameter tend to compress the brain and compromise blood supply and cerebrospinal fluid (CSF) flow.

Case 32

1 **False** Characteristically, the degenerative loss affects upper and lower motor neurones.
2 **False** The condition is usually sporadic. The condition is transmitted in an autosomal dominant fashion in fewer than 10% of cases.
3 **False** This does not occur in motor neurone disease. The nerve supply to the extraocular muscles remains entirely intact.
4 **False** The nerves responsible for urinary and faecal continence remain intact.
5 **False** The primary motor cortex lies immediately in front of the precentral sulcus and is therefore located in the frontal lobe.

Case 33

1 **True** The Arnold–Chiari malformation brings the cerebellar tonsils down to lie in the posterior aspect of the foramen magnum. This tends to transmit increased cerebrospinal fluid (CSF) pressure during a Valsalva's manoeuvre into the central canal instead of the spinal CSF.
2 **True** Sudden extension of the slit-like dissections or central canal enlargement can occur in some patients following a cough or sneeze.
3 **False** Contraction of the detrusor muscle in response to activation of the bladder stretch reflex is parasympathetic. However, the nerve supply from the hypogastric plexus to the urethral sphincter mechanism is sympathetic.
4 **True** The reflex arc that controls

micturition is at the level of the S3 nerve root and S3 segment of the cord. It is therefore able to continue to operate after various lesions of the nervous system, such as spinal cord compression.
5 **False** Micturition itself involves complete volitional relaxation of the external sphincter and relaxation of the pelvic floor.

Case 34

1 **False** Facial sensation is mediated by the Vth nerve and the C2 nerve root over the angle of the mandible.
2 **False** It extends to the vertex (the uppermost point of the head on forward gaze).
3 **True** Schwann cell membranes are extensively coiled around the axon to form a thick myelin sheath.
4 **False** Corneal sensation is mediated by the ophthalmic division of the trigeminal nerve.
5 **False** The innervation to this region is derived from C2 and C3.

Case 35

1 **False** It is one of the branches of the sciatic nerve.
2 **True** Pressure damage, particularly of the part overlying the head of the fibula, is the most frequent type of injury.
3 **True** Sarcoidosis, amyloidosis and causes of nerve ischaemia, such as cryoglobulinaemia, Sjögren's syndrome, Wegener's granulomatosis and systemic sclerosis, are also sometimes implicated in mononeuritis multiplex.
4 **True** Weakness of the peroneal and anterior tibial muscles can occur in facioscapulohumeral muscular dystrophy.
5 **True** Involvement of the lateral femoral cutaneous nerve results in pain in this area.

Case 36

1 **True** Unless the brain stem is also damaged, compensatory mechanisms rapidly come into play.
2 **True** The weak vestibular apparatus is unable to 'push' the eyes to the opposite side. The direction of nystagmus is away from the side of the lesion.
3 **True** Unilateral damage to the cerebellum prevents it 'drawing' the eyes to the same side. The direction of nystagmus is towards the side of the lesion.
4 **False** Ataxic nystagmus is a pattern of nystagmus produced characteristically by demyelinating lesions affecting the medial longitudinal fasciculus—the nerve fibre bundle connecting the IIIrd, IVth and VIth cranial nerve nuclei in the brain stem.
5 **False** The vertebrobasilar arterial supply is more likely to be implicated.

Case 37

1 **False** Both of these conditions can cause ptosis.
2 **False** The sympathetic pathway does not run in the internal capsule.
3 **False** In Horner's syndrome, sympathetic denervation leaves the pupil constricted. If ambient light is low, the normal pupil on the other side will be dilated and the difference between the two becomes easier to see.
4 **False** The facial nerve (VIIth cranial nerve) closes the eye. A facial nerve palsy (Bell's palsy) does not cause ptosis.
5 **True** Demyelination of the dorsolateral brain stem can involve descending sympathetic nerve fibres.

Case 38

1 **True** Not all types of myotonic syndrome behave in this way, but reduced myotonia

on warm up is true of myotonic dystrophy and Thomsen's disease.
2 **True** The mutation underlying myotonic dystrophy is caused by a trinucleotide repeat expansion that exhibits anticipation — the manifestations of the disease become worse and occur earlier in life in successive generations.
3 **True** This is one of the features that distinguishes myotonic dystrophy from myotonia congenita (Thomsen's disease) in which muscle power, particularly in early life, tends to be increased.
4 **True** Testicular atrophy with azoospermia and erectile dysfunction is a characteristic feature of the condition.
5 **False** Frontal balding and ptosis are associated with myotonic dystrophy, but lenticular involvement is through cataract formation.

Case 39

1 **True** The opposite is much less certain, and it seems likely that, when it does appear to have occurred, reinfection with chicken pox has led to reactivation of latent infection.
2 **True** Young children who present with what appears to be recurrent otitis can be 'cured' using an antireflux regimen.
3 **True** The herpes zoster virus has a double-stranded DNA core of around 80 million base pairs.
4 **False** This serious complication of chicken pox appears 3–5 days into the course of the illness in up to 20% of adults. The symptoms of dyspnoea, fever, tachypnoea and cough are associated with pleuritic chest pain, haemoptysis and sometimes cyanosis.
5 **False** In Ramsay–Hunt syndrome, the geniculate ganglion of the facial nerve is involved.

Case 40

1 **True** The clinical phenotypes include foot deformities, progressive distal muscle atrophy and weakness, gait abnormalities, absent reflexes and sensory impairment.
2 **True** It is an autosomal dominant demyelinating polyneuropathy which results from duplications or point mutations of the gene for 'peripheral myelin protein 22' on chromosome 17p11.2-p12.
3 **True** In paraneoplastic sensory neuropathy, autoantibodies to neuronal antigens have become useful diagnostic markers for an underlying carcinoma, especially anti-Hu antibodies. Strong circumstantial evidence suggests that the autoimmune response that leads to the formation of these antibodies may be responsible for the pathogenesis of some of these neuropathic syndromes.
4 **True** Delay in motor development stages, particularly walking, is a relatively common presentation.
5 **False** Patients usually live a normal lifespan and are not usually disabled to the point of immobility.

Case 41

1 **True** Bleeding from arteriovenous malformations is also relatively common.
2 **True** In this 5%, almost one in three have multiple aneurysms, often at the junction of the posterior communicating artery and the internal carotid artery or the junction of the anterior communicating and anterior cerebral arteries.
3 **False** The death rate at 24 h is 25% and this rises to 50% at 3 months.
4 **True** Fortunately, the annual risk of rupture of berry aneurysms is low.
5 **False** Pinpoint pupils are characteristic, associated with impairment of doll's eyes movements, hypertension and frequently

hyperpyrexia, leading to death within a few hours.

Case 42

1 **False** All components of the nervous system can be affected.
2 **False** The diffuse involvement of the paraventricular region of the hypothalamus around the third ventricle affects the paraventricular nuclei, the supraoptic nuclei and the suprachiasmatic nuclei.
3 **False** Involvement of the facial nerve is relatively common, but the problem is usually unilateral and tends to resolve promptly.
4 **True** The olfactory nerves lie immediately beneath the medial part of the frontal lobes.
5 **True** Such a presentation is unusual, but well described.

Case 43

1 **False** Both are very unusual in this condition.
2 **False** The cause of the condition remains unknown.
3 **True** Although most organs of the body are affected, significant clinical involvement of most organs, other than the lungs, skin (25% of cases), eyes (25% of cases) and lymph nodes (77–90% of cases), is rare.
4 **True** The cytokines produced by T-helper type 1 cells are heavily implicated in inducing granulomatous tissue reactions.
5 **True** Of these, one in seven is caused by sarcoidosis.

Case 44

1 **False** The airflow shifted with each breath during quiet respiration is the tidal volume.
2 **False** The volume of air in the conducting airways between the mouth and respiratory bronchioles that have no gas exchange capability constitutes the anatomical 'dead space'. The air remaining within the lungs after a quiet exhalation is the 'functional residual capacity'.
3 **False** The composition of air is 21% oxygen, 78% nitrogen, 0.04% carbon dioxide and 0.92% other constituents.
4 **False** The normal resting respiratory rate is closer to 12–15 breaths per minute.
5 **True** A classical restrictive pattern is characterized by a decrease in vital capacity with a normal forced expiratory volume in 1 s to forced vital capacity (FEV1/FVC) ratio.

Case 45

1 **True** In about 60% of adults, pain and stiffness in the back, radiating to the buttock and posterior thigh, are typical. Particularly in children and adolescents, the first sign may be arthritis of the hip or knee.
2 **False** It is a rare complication of psoriasis, much less common than rheumatoid arthritis-like synovitis complicated in 20% of cases by involvement of the sacroiliac joints and sometimes by ankylosing spondylitis.
3 **False** Surprisingly, the process is not usually painful. Links have been drawn with diabetes mellitus and other neuropathic conditions, although there is no gross neurological deficit.
4 **False** Compared with HLA-B27-negative individuals, the chances are very high, but they only amount to 5% of men and 0.6% of women.
5 **True** So are patients with Reiter's disease and psoriasis.

Case 46

1 **True** A proportion of cases terminate in myelofibrosis or acute myeloid leukaemia.
2 **True** This patient demonstrated one of the most common complications.
3 **True** Significant reductions in red cell size

are unusual in thyrotoxicosis. Macrocytosis in hypothyroidism is a more useful sign, but again it is a late sign.
4 **False** The usual features of hyperviscosity are related to disturbances of cerebral circulation. Typically, they include dizziness, headaches, tinnitus, vertigo and rushing in the ears.
5 **False** Sustained hypoxia does cause polycythaemia, but right to left shunts carrying deoxygenated blood into the systemic circulation (rather than left to right shunts) are required for polycythaemia to develop.

Case 47

1 **True** It occurs in around 0.1% of the population, and is transmitted in an autosomal dominant fashion.
2 **True** It raises the level of von Willebrand's factor.
3 **False** Platelet and vessel wall disorders tend to produce bleeding into the skin, mucous membranes or the gastrointestinal or genitourinary tracts immediately after trauma. Patients with coagulation disorders bleed into deep subcutaneous tissues, muscles, joints or body cavities hours or days later.
4 **False** von Willebrand's factor, although reduced in patients with von Willebrand's disease, is an acute phase protein and can reach almost normal levels during systemic inflammation, pregnancy and some central nervous system disorders.
5 **True** Splenomegaly predisposes to the splenic sequestration of platelets.

Case 48

1 **True** Radiofrequency ablation of the abnormal conducting bundle results in cure.
2 **True** Q waves in the same leads suggest a right-sided aberrant pathway.
3 **True** An anomalous conducting pathway is

either used or not used. Intuitively, dysrhythmias driven by conduction anomalies will start and end abruptly. A gradual return to normality occurs in anxiety and other causes of norepinephrine or epinephrine excess, such as phaeochromocytoma.
4 **False** The potential is predominantly generated by a potassium ion gradient.
5 **False** In myocardial cells that exhibit automaticity, the resting potential decreases spontaneously towards the threshold potential at which a full depolarizing ion flux occurs.

Case 49

1 **True** When the narrowing is above the ductus arteriosus, the latter usually remains patent in postnatal life. Coarctation is associated with 5% of patients with congenital heart disease overall.
2 **False** The ductus arteriosis provides a shunt from the right ventricle to the aortic arch and systemic circulation.
3 **True** Coarctation is also associated with intracranial berry aneurysms.
4 **True** About 60% of patients have no symptoms. Cerebrovascular accidents, bacterial endocarditis and symptoms (nominally) associated with hypertension and intermittent claudication are typical in the remainder.
5 **True** The collateral circulation is associated with bruits.

Case 50

1 **False** The septum secundum grows down to overlap the ostium secundum on the right side, leaving the septum primum to act as a flap valve allowing a right to left atrial shunt.
2 **True** In about 20% of adults, it is possible to pass a probe from the right to the left atrium *in vivo*.
3 **True** The remaining defects being

pulmonary stenosis, right ventricular hypertrophy and a medially displaced (overriding) aorta.
4 **False** This truncoconal septum divides the common, primitive outflow vessel from the heart into the pulmonary artery and the aorta. Defects in its development can lead to transposition of the great vessels or persistent truncus arteriosus. The atria are divided by the septum primum and the septum secundum.
5 **True** The mechanisms include increased pulmonary blood flow and blood pressure, hypoxia, acidosis and polycythaemia.

Index

Note:
Index entries on pages 135–147 refer to the answers of the MCQs, but index references are only included if information is provided that is not discussed in the case history.
Page numbers in **bold** refer to the diagnosis and main features of the case history.

abdominal pain
    acute intermittent porphyria **31–3**, 137–8
    carcinoid syndrome **73–5**, 141
    intermittent, in renal tubular acidosis **37–9**, 138
acanthosis nigricans 52
acidosis *see* metabolic acidosis
acids
    decreased excretion 38
    increased ingestion/production 38, 138
acquired immunodeficiency (AIDS) dementia complex **1–3**, 135
acromegaly 66
ACTH (adrenocorticotrophic hormone)
    elevation in Cushing's disease 68, 69
    Synacthen test 50, 58
Addison's disease **49–51**, 139
    classic features 50, 51, 139
adrenal cortex 70
    autoimmune destruction 50
    steroid hormone biosynthesis 69, 70, 141
adrenal preandrogens 69, 141
AIDS dementia complex **1–3**, 135
aldose reductase inhibitors 92
aldosterone 36
alkali, loss, acidosis due to 38–9
alkaline phosphatase, raised level
    carcinoid syndrome 73
    Paget's disease of bone 137
    primary biliary cirrhosis 78
    Wilson's disease 81
amine precursor uptake and decarboxylation (APUD) cells 24
δ-aminolaevulinic acid, synthesis 32
amyotrophic lateral sclerosis 86, 142
anaemia
    megaloblastic 121
    normochromic, normocytic 35
anatomical 'dead space' 116, 145
androgens, deficiency 56
aneurysms
    giant **108–10**, 144–5
    infective (mycotic) 109
    risk of rupture and death rate 109, 110, 144
    saccular (berry) 109, 110, 144, 146
angina pectoris 7

angioid streaks 14
anion gap 39
    calculation 38
    normal range 39, 138
ankylosing spondylitis, HLA-B27 and 118, 145
ankylosis, joints 118
anterior horn cells, degenerative loss 86
antiandrogens 57
anticholinergic drugs 11, 136
anticipation, genetic 144
anti-Hu antibodies 106
antimitochondrial antibodies 78
antineoplastic agents 5
antineutrophil cytoplasmic antibodies (ANCAs) 15, 16, 17, 136
aorta, coarctation **129–30**, 146
aortic arch, development 130
APUD cells 24
Arnold–Chiari malformation 88, 89, 142
arteriovenous malformations, bleeding 109, 144
arthritis mutilans **118–19**, 145
aspirin, brain stem stroke 97
asthma, Churg–Strauss disease and 17, 136
ataxic nystagmus 143
atherosclerosis 97
atrial septal defects 9, 132, 146
atrial septum
    abnormalities 132, 146
    formation 132
atrioventricular septal defects 131
autoimmune diseases 59
    risk in Addison's disease 51, 139
autoimmune thyrotoxicosis **46–8**, 139
autoimmunity 59
axonal degeneration 93

backache/back pain
    primary biliary cirrhosis 78
    spinal tuberculosis 7
    syringomyelia 87
Becker's disease **100–1**
behaviour
    AIDS dementia complex **1–3**, 135
    change in frontal lobe meningioma **83–4**, 142
Bell's palsy 93, 102, 143
Berger's disease (IgA nephropathy) **34–6**, 138
bile 79
bile acids/salts 53, 79
    oral administration 79
    pool, enterohepatic recirculation 79, 80, 142
    reabsorption 79, 142
bile pigments 33, 138
bilirubin, elevation in Wilson's disease 81

bisphosphonates, Paget's disease 26
bladder, neural control 88–9, 142–3
bleeding, reduction in von Willebrand's factor 123
bleeding diathesis 123
bleeding time 125
blood–brain barrier 72
blood vessel walls, disorders 76, 77, 125, 141, 146
blood viscosity, increased 121
B lymphocytes 59, 140
bone
   formation and composition 26, 137
   growth 26
   remodelling 25, 26
bowel control 88–9, 142–3
   loss 87–9
bradycardia, sinus, causes 10–11, 135–6
brain, anchoring to skull 71, 72, 141
brain stem
   cerebrovascular accident **94–5**, 143
   decompensation 95
   lesions 97
   stroke **96–8**, 143
brain tumours 83–4
   metastatic 83, 142
   primary 83
breast, development 56
breast cancer 4
   metastatic **18–20**, 136
   occult intraductal 19
   oestrogen receptor-expressing 19, 136
   risk factors 18–19, 20, 136
breathlessness
   Eisenmenger's syndrome **131–3**, 146–7
   idiopathic fibrosing alveolitis **116–17**, 145
   pulmonary sarcoidosis **114–15**, 145
   spinal tuberculosis 7
Broca's area 109
Brown-Séquard syndrome 8
bruising
   Cushing's disease 68
   von Willebrand's disease 123
bruits, coarctation of aorta 130
bulbar palsy 5, 6, 86, 135

café-au-lait patches 22, 136
calcitonin, as tumour marker 20
calcium
   low circulating levels 41, 138
   urinary 38
cancer
   hereditary syndromes 20
   mechanisms and aetiological factors 19–20
   peripheral neuropathy differential diagnosis 106, 144
   see also breast cancer; testicular cancer
carcinoembryonic antigen (CEA) 20, 136
carcinoid syndrome **73–5**, 141
carcinoid tumours 74
   hepatic metastases 74, 75, 141
cardiac anomalies
   atrial septal defects 9, 132, 146
   coarctation of aorta 130

   congenital, cyanotic 132
   Eisenmenger's syndrome **131–3**, 146–7
   Shprintzen's syndrome 9–11, 135–6
cardiac cells
   depolarization 127
   resting potential 127, 128, 146
cataracts 144
cauda equina damage 89
CD4+ T-helper cells, HIV receptor 2, 135
cell-mediated immunity 140
   inhibition by cortisol 50
central nervous system, development 44
cephalothoracic lipodystrophy 53
cerebellar degeneration, subacute 5
cerebellar disease, nystagmus 95, 143
cerebellar tonsils 88, 142
cerebral circulation, hyperviscosity features 121, 146
cerebral sarcoidosis **111–13**, 145
cerebral venous sinuses 71, 141
cerebrospinal fluid (CSF) 71–2
   absorption by arachnoid villi 72, 141
   composition 71–2, 141
   functions and synthesis 71, 72, 141
   obstruction by haemangioblastoma 88
   outflow obstruction, giant aneurysms 108
   persistent leak **71–2**, 141
   pressure increase 88, 142
cerebrovascular accidents
   brain stem **94–5**, 143
   coarctation of aorta and 146
ceruloplasmin 81, 82, 142
cervicogenic otalgia 103
Charcot–Marie–Tooth disease 105–6
   symptoms and signs 106, 144
chemosis 47, 139
chest infections, pain referred to ears 103
chest pain, exercise-induced 7
chicken pox 103
chloride, resorption increase 38
choking, motor neurone disease **85–6**
cholangitis, diffuse non-suppurative 78, 141
cholecystitis 79
cholecystokinin 79
cholesterol gallstones 79
chondrodystrophic myotonia 101
choroid plexus, CSF synthesis 71, 141
chromosomal disorders 10
chronic obstructive pulmonary disease (COPD) 133, 147
Churg–Strauss disease 16
   asthma association 17, 136
Chvostek's sign 41
cirrhosis
   primary biliary **78–80**, 141–2
   Wilson's disease 81
clotting disorders 125
clumsiness 87
coagulation disorders 125, 146
coarctation of aorta **129–30**, 146
collagen, in bone 26, 137
'collapse', in recurrent paraganglioma **23–4**, 137

colour vision, desaturation 47
common bile duct, dilatation 79
common peroneal nerve 93
   diabetic mononeuropathy affecting **92–3**, 143
   pressure damage 93
congenital adrenal hyperplasia 70, 141
congenital heart disease, cyanotic 132
connective tissues 13
   inherited disorders 13
convulsions
   cerebral sarcoidosis 111
   grand mal 60
copper
   accumulation 82, 142
   excretion 82
   metabolism and sources 82
   serum levels in Wilson's disease 81, 142
corneal reflex 91
corneal sensation 143
corona radiata 86
coronary heart disease, rare in lipodystrophy 139
'corticobulbar' fibres 86
corticospinal tracts 86
   decussation 135
cortisol 70
   Addison's disease 50
   Cushing's disease 68
   excretion 70, 141
   functions 50
   increased levels 70, 140–1
   production, defective 70, 141
   stress response 51, 70, 139
C peptide 61, 140
cramps, in pseudohypoparathyroidism 41
creatine kinase, elevated levels 4, 5, 6
creatinine, in IgA nephropathy 34
Crohn's disease 118
Cryptosporidium parvum 3
c-src gene 26, 137
Cushing's disease (pituitary-dependent Cushing's
   syndrome) **68–70**, 140–1
cutis laxa 14
cyanosis, Eisenmenger's syndrome **131–3**, 146–7
cyclic AMP (cAMP), urinary excretion 41, 42
cytokines, sarcoid granulomas 115, 145

DDAVP (1-desamino-8-D-arginine vasopressin)
   125, 146
deafness *see* hearing loss
defaecation, control 89
dehydrogenases 75
dementia, in AIDS **1–3**, 135
demyelinating polyneuropathy 106, 144
demyelination 93, 143
dentition defects, in pseudohypoparathyroidism
   41, 42, 138
dermatomyositis **4–6**, 135
detrusor muscle contraction 142
dexamethasone suppression test 68
diabetes insipidus
   central 29
   cerebral sarcoidosis 111

   Langerhans cell histiocytosis 29, 137
   postoperative 137
diabetes mellitus
   acquired partial lipodystrophy **52–4**, 139
   risk in Addison's disease 51, 139
diabetic ketoacidosis 38
diabetic mononeuropathy **92–3**, 143
diarrhoea, carcinoid syndrome 73
diplopia
   autoimmune thyrotoxicosis 47
   causes 47
   metastatic breast cancer **18–20**, 136
disseminated intravascular coagulation 141
dizziness **94–5**, 143
dopamine 56
   agonists and antagonists 56
double vision *see* diplopia
Down's syndrome 10
ductus arteriosus 146
   coarctation of aorta site 130, 146
   patent 130
Dunnigan–Kobberling syndrome 53
duodenal ulceration 120
dysarthria, Wilson's disease **81–2**, 142
dysphagia, motor neurone disease 85

ear pain
   acute **15–17**, 136
   causes 103
   Ramsay–Hunt syndrome **102–4**, 144
eating, 'funny feelings' relieved by 60, 62, 140
Eaton–Lambert syndrome 5
ectopia lentis 13
Edwards' syndrome 10
Ehlers–Danlos syndrome 14
Eisenmenger's syndrome **131–3**, 146–7
elastic fibres, disorders 14
electrocardiogram (ECG) 73–4, 126–7
electromyography, motor neurone disease 85
embryology
   aortic arch 130
   CNS, thyroid hormone role 44
   heart 132
   neural crest 22, 136–7
   thyroid gland 44, 138
enophthalmos 97
epidermolysis bullosa 14
epilepsy, intracranial tumours 83, 142
epiphyseal plate and epiphyses 26
epistaxis **15–17**, 76, 136
erectile dysfunction 63
   primary hypopituitarism **58–9**, 140
erythroblasts 121
erythrocyte sedimentation rate (ESR) 16
erythropoiesis 121
exophthalmos, Langerhans cell histiocytosis 29
extraocular muscles
   motor neurone disease 142
   palsies 47–8, 139
eyelid
   drooping **96–8**, 143
   lid lag 47, 48, 139

retraction 47
eye movements, conjugate 47, 139
eye muscles, palsies 47–8, 139
eyes, swelling around 46–7, 139

facial flushing, carcinoid syndrome 73–5, 141
facial nerve
   cerebral sarcoidosis 113, 145
   herpes zoster infection 102, 144
   palsy 143
facial sensation 91, 143
facial sensory loss 90–1, 143
facial weakness, Ramsay–Hunt syndrome 102–4, 144
facies
   pseudohypoparathyroidism 41
   Shprintzen's syndrome 9–11
faecal continence 142
fasciculations 85
fat
   absorption 53
   malabsorption 78–9
   metabolism abnormality in lipodystrophy 52, 54, 139
fat (body), loss in lipodystrophy 52
fatigue *see* tiredness
α-fetoprotein, hepatocellular carcinoma 20, 136
fibrillin 13
fibrosing alveolitis, idiopathic 116–17, 145
finger clubbing, idiopathic fibrosing alveolitis 116
flavin adenine dinucleotide (FAD) 74, 141
follicle-stimulating hormone (FSH) 55, 140
foot deformity, Charcot–Marie–Tooth disease 106, 144
foot drop 92, 93
foramen caecum 44, 138
frontal balding 144
frontal lobe
   lesions, micturition control loss 89
   meningioma 83–4, 142
functional residual capacity 116, 145

galactorrhoea 57, 139
gall-bladder pain 79
gallstones 79
   asymptomatic 142
gas exchange 116
gastrointestinal bleeding, recurrent 123–5, 146
gastro-oesophageal reflux 103, 104
geniculate ganglion, herpes zoster infection 102, 144
genome 64
giant aneurysms 108–10, 144–5
giant-cell (temporal) arteritis 16
gibbus 7, 76
gigantism 65–7, 140
giggling, frontal lobe meningioma 83–4, 142
glomerulonephritis
   chronic renal failure in 35
   IgA nephropathy 34–6, 138
   rapidly progressive crescentic 15–16
glucagon 62

intramuscular injection 62, 140
glucocorticoids 50, 69–70
   functions 50
   replacement in Addison's disease 51, 139
   synthesis 70
glucose
   elevated blood levels 94
   tubular reabsorption 36
glycerol 53
goitre, appearance in pseudohypoparathyroidism 40–2, 138
G protein-coupled receptors 41–2, 138
G protein mutations
   McCune–Albright syndrome 42
   pseudohypoparathyroidism 41
grand mal convulsion 60
granuloma, sarcoid 115
granulomatosis, Wegener's 15–17, 136
Graves' disease (autoimmune thyrotoxicosis) 46–8, 139
   eye disease 46–8, 139
growth
   accelerated in lipodystrophy 52
   after birth 66, 140
   catch-up and 'catch-down' 140
   prepubertal 66, 140
   retardation, primary hypothyroidism 43, 45, 139
growth hormone
   deficiency 66
   raised levels 66
growth hormone-secreting adenoma 65–7, 140
GTPases 41–2, 138
   activation 41–2, 138
   subunits 41–2, 138
guanosine triphosphate (GTP), hydrolysis 41, 138
guanosine triphosphate (GTP)-binding proteins *see* GTPases
Guillain–Barré syndrome 6, 106
gum, lesion in Langerhans cell histiocytosis 28–9, 137
gynaecomastia 55, 56, 64
   differential diagnosis 56

haem
   biosynthesis 32
   biosynthesis defects 31, 32, 137–8
   catabolism 33, 137
haemangioblastoma 87–8, 142–3
haematemesis
   brain stem cerebrovascular accident 94–5, 143
   hereditary haemorrhagic telangiectases 76–7, 141
haemoglobin, raised levels 120
haemolytic uraemic syndrome 77
hands, stiffness in pseudohypoparathyroidism 40–2, 138
headache
   cranial Paget's disease 25
   intracranial tumours 83
   macroprolactinoma 55–7, 139
   pituitary macroadenoma 71

hearing loss
  cranial Paget's disease **25–7**, 137
  progressive, in Wegener's granulomatosis 15
  Wegener's granulomatosis 15
heart
  conduction defects 127, 146
  embryology 132
  murmurs, in carcinoid syndrome 75, 141
  rate, control 11, 135
  see also cardiac anomalies
height 66
  congenital hypothyroidism 43, 45, 139
  gigantism 65
Henoch–Schönlein purpura 35, 77
hepatitis B, HBsAg 17, 136
hepatocellular carcinoma, α-fetoprotein 20, 136
hepatomegaly, in carcinoid syndrome 75, 141
hereditary haemorrhagic telangiectases **76–7**, 141
herpes zoster 90, 91, 93, 103
  Ramsay–Hunt syndrome 102–4, 144
  reactivation 103
herpes zoster virus 103, 144
hirsutism, Cushing's disease 68
histiocytic cells (foam cells) 28
histiocytosis X (Langerhans cell histiocytosis) **28–30**, 137
  classic features 29, 30, 137
HIV (human immunodeficiency virus) 2, 135
HIV infection
  Kaposi's sarcoma 136
  memory loss and abnormal behaviour **1–3**, 135
hormones, ectopic production 24
Horner's syndrome 76, 96, 143
  causes 97
human chorionic gonadotrophin (hCG) 20, 136
hydrogen ions, excretion failure 38, 138
hydroxyapatite 26, 137
5-hydroxyindoleacetic acid (5-HIAA) 73, 141
  formation 74
17-hydroxyprogesterone 70, 141
5-hydroxytryptamine (5-HT), excess secretion 74, 141
hypercalcaemia, in malignancy 20, 136
hypercalciuria, hereditary idiopathic **37–9**, 138
hypercholesterolaemia 139
hypercortisolaemia 70, 140–1
hyperkalaemia 38
  Addison's disease 50, 139
hypermetabolic syndromes 139
hypermetabolism 53
hyperpnoea 116
hypersensitivity 59
hypertension
  pulmonary *see* pulmonary hypertension
  refractory **129–30**, 146
hypertriglyceridaemia 53
  chronic renal failure 35
  lipodystrophy association 52, 53, 139
  secondary, causes 53
hyperviscosity 121, 146
hypoadrenalism 58

hypoadrenocorticism, primary (Addison's disease) **49–51**, 139
hypoandrogenaemia 64
hypogastric plexus 89, 142
hypoglycaemic coma 62, 140
hypogonadism
  hypogonadotrophic *see* hypogonadotrophic hypogonadism
  myotonic dystrophy 100, 144
  primary, in Klinefelter's syndrome 140
  progressive secondary 58
hypogonadotrophic hypogonadism
  differential diagnosis 59
  growth hormone-secreting adenoma causing 140
hyponatraemia, Addison's disease 50, 139
hypopituitarism, primary **58–9**, 140
hypotension, Addison's disease 139
hypothalamus, paraventricular region 113, 145
hypothyroidism
  causes 44
  congenital 43, 45, 138–9
  facial appearance 43, 45
  macrocytosis 146
  primary **43–5**, 49, 138–9, 140
  secondary to pituitary failure 59, 140
hypoxia, sustained, secondary polycythaemia after 121, 146

immune complexes, deposition 16, 136
immune surveillance, blood–brain barrier and 72
immune system-mediated diseases 59
immune tolerance 59, 140
immunodeficiency 59
immunoglobulin, monoclonal, as tumour marker 20
immunoglobulin A (IgA) 35
  deposition 35, 77, 138
immunoglobulin A (IgA) nephropathy **34–6**, 138
infections, acquired partial lipodystrophy after 52, 138
inflammatory bowel disease, ankylosing spondarthropathies 118, 145
insulin 61
  first pass metabolism 61, 140
  metabolic effects 61–2
  resistance, lipodystrophy association 52, 139
  secretion 61
insulinoma **60–2**, 140
  incidence 61, 140
interventricular septum
  abnormalities 132
  formation 132
intervertebral disc herniation 8
intracranial haemorrhage 109
intracranial tumours 83
  growth rate 83, 142
  neurofibromatosis 21–2, 136
iodine
  maternal deficiency 44
  sources 45, 139
iron deficiency 121
ischaemia, peripheral 120, 121, 122, 146

itching
  perception 79
  primary biliary cirrhosis 78–80, 142

jaundice
  primary biliary cirrhosis 78, 142
  Wilson's disease 81–2, 142
jaw, angle, sensory loss 91, 143
jaw bone, destruction, Langerhans cell histiocytosis 28–9, 137
joints, laxity 14

Kaposi's sarcoma 136
Kayser–Fleischer rings 81, 82, 142
ketoacidosis 38
kidney, function 35–6
Klinefelter's syndrome 10, **63–4**, 140
kyphosis 7–8, 76

lactate dehydrogenase 4
lactation 56
lactic acidosis 38
lagophthalmos 47, 48, 139
Langerhans cell histiocytosis **28–30**, 137
lateral femoral cutaneous nerve, damage 93, 143
Lawrence syndrome 53
leg
  growth 66, 140
  loss of pain sensation 87
  muscle wasting 105
  soft tissue sarcoma **12–14**, 136
lentiviruses 2
lethargy
  Addison's disease 49
  IgA nephropathy **34–6**, 138
  see also tiredness
leucocytosis 120
leukemia, polycythaemia rubra vera association 120, 145
libido, loss, in macroprolactinoma **55–7**, 139
lid lag 47, 48, 139
lid retraction 47
limb, growth 66, 140
lipase, pancreatic 53
lipodystrophy 52–3
  acquired partial **52–4**, 139
  cephalothoracic 53
  types 53
liver
  fatty 53
  metastases, carcinoid tumours 74, 75, 141
liver biopsy, sarcoid granulomas 115, 145
lower motor neurones
  degenerative loss 86, 142
  paralysis 135
lumbosacral dural ectasia 13
lung, opacification 114
lung disease, restrictive, pattern 116, 117, 145
luteinizing hormone (LH) 140
lymphadenopathy, bilateral hilar 115

macrocytosis 146
  differential diagnosis 121

macroprolactinoma **55–7**, 139
  persistent CSF leak after surgery **71–2**, 141
magnetic resonance imaging (MRI), syringomyelia 87–8
Mallory–Weiss tear 94
mandible, lesion in Langerhans cell histiocytosis 28–9, 137
Marcus Gunn pupil 47
Marfan's syndrome 13–14, 130
  mutations causing 136
  prevalence and inheritance 14, 136
  skeletal deformities 136
McCune–Albright syndrome 42
meiosis 64, 140
memory impairment/loss
  HIV infection **1–3**, 135
  Klinefelter's syndrome 63
meningioma, frontal lobe **83–4**, 142
meralgia paraesthetica 93, 143
mesangial IgA disease (IgA nephropathy) **34–6**, 138
mesencephalon 22, 137
metabolic acidosis 38
  anion gap in 39, 138
  causes and types 38
  chronic renal failure 35, 38, 39, 138
  renal tubular 37–8
metastases
  brain 83, 142
  hepatic, in carcinoid tumours 74, 75, 141
microcytosis 122, 145–6
  differential diagnosis 121
microprolactinoma 56
micturition 143
  control 88–9, 142–3
  voluntary inhibition 89
midbrain, development 22, 137
migraine, pain referred to ears 103
miosis (pupillary constriction) 96, 143
mitral regurgitation, Shprintzen's syndrome 9
monoclonal immunoglobulin, as tumour marker 20
mononeuritis multiplex 93, 143
mononeuropathy 93
  diabetic **92–3**, 143
mood, glucocorticoids affecting 50
mosaicism, Klinefelter's syndrome 63, 140
motor cortex 86, 142
motor development, delay 144
motor function 86
motor neurone disease 6, **85–6**, 142
multiple endocrine neoplasia 24
  type 1 137
  type 2a and type 2b 24, 137
multiple sclerosis, Horner's syndrome 98
muscle cell, atrophy 86
muscle power, myotonic dystrophy 100, 144
muscle wasting
  myotonic dystrophy 100
  peroneal muscular atrophy **105–7**, 144
muscle weakness
  dermatomyositis 4, 5, 135
  motor neurone disease 85

myotonic dystrophy 99, 100
  peroneal muscular atrophy **105–7**, 144
  progressive, in Cushing's disease 68
musculocutaneous nerve 93
mutations 64
  types 64
myelin 91, 143
  gene mutations 106
myelomeningocoele 22
myotonia 100
  diseases and forms 100–1
myotonia congenita 100
myotonic dystrophy **99–101**, 143–4
  inheritance 101, 144

NAD+ 75
nasal discharge, persistent CSF leak **71–2**, 141
nausea
  IgA nephropathy **34–6**, 138
  renal tubular acidosis 37
neck, swelling in pseudohypoparathyroidism **40–2**, 138
neoplasia *see* cancer
nephrocalcinosis, in renal tubular acidosis **37–9**, 138
neural crest, development 22
neural plate 22
neural tube
  defects 22
  development 22, 136–7
neurofibromatosis **21–2**
  incidence 21, 136
  phaeochromocytoma complicating **21–2**, 136–7
neuroglycopenia 60
neurological problems, HIV infection 2
neuropsychiatric disease 100
niacin 74
nicotinamide 74
nicotinamide adenine dinucleotide (NAD) 74, 141
nicotinic acid 74, 75, 141
  content of foods 75
nicotinic acid equivalents 75
nocturia, Langerhans cell histiocytosis **28–9**, 137
noradrenaline (norepinephrine), excretion in recurrent paraganglioma 23
nose bleeds (epistaxis) **15–17**, 76, 136
nosebrain (rhinencephalon) 112
numbness, brain stem stroke **96–8**, 143
nystagmus 94–5
  brain stem stroke 94–5, **96–8**, 143
  causes 95
  cerebellar 95, 143
  congenital 95
  'direction of' 95, 143
  optokinetic 95

obesity, Cushing's disease 68
oculomotor nerve (IIIrd cranial nerve), palsy 97, 143
  metastatic breast cancer **18–20**, 136
Oddi, sphincter 79
oedema
  non-pitting, hypothyroidism 45

  periorbital 46–7, 139
oestrogen
  breast development 56
  increased production 56
  receptor, breast cancer 19, 136
olfaction 112–13
olfactory bulb 112
olfactory hallucination **111–13**, 145
olfactory nerves 113, 145
onycholysis 45, 139
optic chiasm, macroprolactinoma affecting 55
Osler–Rendu–Weber disease **76–7**, 141
osmolality, serum 29
osteoblasts and osteoclasts 26
osteomyelitis, spinal, tuberculous 8, 135
osteosarcoma, risk in Paget's disease of bone 137
ostium primum 9, 132, 146
ostium secundum 132, 146
otalgia
  psychogenic 103
  referred 103
oxidases 75
oxidation–reduction reactions 74–5
oxytocin 56

Paget's disease of bone 25
  asymptomatic 27, 137
  cranial **25–7**, 137
pain
  chest, exercise-induced 7
  gall-bladder 79
  loss of sensation 87
  thigh **18–20**, 136
  see also abdominal pain; ear pain
palpitations
  abrupt cessation 127
  causes 127
  episodic **126–8**, 146
  phaeochromocytoma **21–2**
  Shprintzen's syndrome **9–11**, 135–6
panarteritis 16
Pancoast's syndrome 97
pancreatic angiography 60–1
papilloedema, bilateral, in giant aneurysm 108
paraganglioma, recurrent **23–4**, 137
paramyotonia congenita 101
paraneoplastic sensory neuropathy 106, 144
paraneoplastic syndromes 5
parasympathetic system
  bladder innervation 89, 142
  resting heart rate control 11, 135
parathyroid hormone (PTH) 36
  action/functions 41
  elevated levels 138
parathyroid hormone-related peptide (PTHRP) 20, 136
Patau's syndrome 10
pellagra 74–5
penicillamine 81, 82, 142
pericarditis, in tuberculosis 8
periorbital oedema 46–7, 139
peripheral nerves, neuromas 22, 136
peripheral neuropathy 106

peritonitis, in tuberculosis 8
peroneal muscles, wasting 105
peroneal muscular atrophy **105–7**, 144
phaeochromocytoma **21–2**, 23–4, **136–7**
    diagnosis and differential diagnosis 137
    extra-adrenal (recurrent paraganglioma) **23–4**, 137
    incidence 24, 137
pharyngeal arch 130
pharyngitis, streptococcal 77, 141
pheromones 113
phosphate, raised levels 41, 138
photosensitive rash 138
pigmentation, skin
    Addison's disease **49–51**, 139
    neurofibromatosis 22, 136
pituitary, anterior
    autoimmune destruction 58–9, 140
    prolactin synthesis 55, 56, 139
pituitary adenoma
    growth hormone-secreting somatotrophic **65–7**, 140
    macroprolactinoma *see* macroprolactinoma
    microprolactinoma 56
pituitary apoplexy 71
pituitary stalk, damage 29
pituitary tumours, visual field loss 57, 139
platelets 125
    counts 123, 125
    production 125
    splenic sequestration 125, 146
    von Willebrand's disease 123
platelet wall disorders 125, 146
pleurisy, in tuberculosis 8
Pneumocystis carinii, in HIV infection 1, 2–3
pneumocytes 116
pneumonia
    Pneumocystis carinii 3
    varicella 103, 104, 144
polyarteritis nodosa 16, 136
polycythaemia
    relative 121
    secondary 121
polycythaemia rubra vera **120–2**, 145–6
polydipsia, psychogenic 137
polyneuropathy
    demyelinating 106, 144
    paraneoplastic 5
    sensorimotor 5
pons, sympathetic pathway 96, 143
pontine haemorrhages 109, 110, 144
porphobilinogen 32
    excretion 138
porphobilinogen deaminase, deficiency 31–2
porphyria
    acute intermittent **31–3**, 137–8
    erythropoietic 32
    hepatic 33
porphyrins 32
potassium
    chronic renal failure 35
    negative potential of myocardial cells 128, 146

    tubular reabsorption 36
    see also hyperkalaemia
Pott's disease **7–8**, 135
pregnancy, hormone levels 56
primary biliary cirrhosis **78–80**, 141–2
proerythroblasts 121
proinsulin 61
prolactin
    functions 56
    macroprolactinoma 55–6, 139
    synthesis 55, 56, 139
proprioception 135
proptosis 46
prostatic-specific antigen 20
protease inhibitors 2, 135
proximal myopathy, Cushing's disease 68, 70, 141
pruritus, primary biliary cirrhosis 78–80, 142
pseudobulbar palsy 5, 86
pseudohypoparathyroidism **40–2**, 138
    inheritance 138
pseudopseudohypoparathyroidism 41
pseudoxanthoma elasticum 14
psoriatic arthritis **118–19**, 145
psychiatric dysfunction, in acute intermittent porphyria 31
psychiatric features, Wilson's disease 82
psychogenic otalgia 103
ptosis 97, 143, 144
puberty, bone growth and 26
pulmonary fibrosis 116–17
    pathology 116
    pulmonary sarcoidosis 114–15, 145
pulmonary hypertension
    COPD 133, 147
    Eisenmenger's syndrome 131
    secondary 132
    Shprintzen's syndrome 9
pulmonary pressure, increased 132
pulmonary sarcoidosis **114–15**, 145
pupillary response 47
pupils
    constriction (miosis) 96, 143
    pinpoint 144
    relative afferent defects 47
purpura
    Henoch–Schönlein 77
    thrombotic thrombocytopenic 77
'pyramidal' tract 86

radiofrequency ablation 127, 146
Ramsay–Hunt syndrome **102–4**, 144
rash
    dermatomyositis **4–6**, 135
    photosensitive, in acute intermittent porphyria 138
    psoriatic arthritis **118–19**, 145
red blood cells, production and volume 121
Reiter's disease 118
renal failure, chronic 35, 38
    IgA nephropathy **34–6**, 138
    metabolic acidosis 35, 38, 39, 138
renal failure, end-stage 35, 138

renal osteodystrophy 35
renal stones, renal tubular acidosis 37–8
renal tubular acidosis **37–9**, 138
    type 1 (distal) 38
    type 2 (proximal) 38
renal tubules, function 35, 36, 138
respiration, external and internal 116
respiratory rate, resting 117, 145
reticulocytes 121
retroviruses 2, 135
rhinencephalon 112
rhombencephalon 22, 137
rib notching 130
right to left shunts 131, 146
Romberg's test 94

sacroiliac joints, spinal tuberculosis 7, 135
sarcoid granulomas 115
sarcoidosis 115
    cerebral **111–13**, 145
    pulmonary **114–15**, 145
sarcoma, soft tissue **12–14**, 136
Schwann cell membranes 91, 143
Schwarts–Jampel syndrome 101
sciatic nerve 143
Seip–Berardinelli syndrome 53
semicircular canal disease, nystagmus due to 95
sensory loss/impairment
    brain stem stroke 96–8, 143
    facial **90–1**, 143
    peroneal muscular atrophy 106, 144
    syringomyelia 87
serum sickness 17
shingles *see* herpes zoster
short stature 66
Shprintzen's syndrome **9–11**, 135–6
sinoatrial node 127, 128, 146
sinus bradycardia, causes 10–11, 135–6
sinusitis, chronic 103
sinus tachycardia, causes 10, 11, 136
skeletal deformities, Marfanoid habitus 136
skin
    dryness in primary hypothyroidism 43
    pigmentation *see* pigmentation
    smoothness in hypopituitarism 58, 59, 140
    thinning 70, 140–1
skull bones, formation 26, 137
skull enlargement in Paget's disease 25
smell, sense of 112–13
    olfactory hallucination **111–13**, 145
smoking, histiocytosis X link 29, 137
sodium, cardiac cell depolarization 127
soft tissue sarcoma **12–14**, 136
somatostatin analogues 79
sorbitol 92
space-occupying lesions 113, 145
spastic paraparesis 8
speech disturbances 5–6
    'Donald Duck like' 6
    giant aneurysm 108–10, 144–5
    slurred, in motor neurone disease **85–6**
spina bifida 22

spinal cord
    ballooning of central cavity 88, 89
    compression 8
    damage, bladder/bowel control loss 89
    hemisection 8
spine
    growth 66, 140
    mid-thoracic, in tuberculosis 8, 135
    tuberculosis 7–8, 135
    tuberculous osteomyelitis 8, 135
spinothalamic fibres 8
splenomegaly 146
spondarthropathies 118, 119
stature 66
    see also height
Steinert's disease (myotonic dystrophy) **99–101**, 143–4
steroid hormone, biosynthesis in adrenal cortex 69, 70, 141
stiffness 101
    psoriatic arthritis **118–19**, 145
streptococcal pharyngitis 77, 141
stress, cortisol response 51, 70, 139
stroke, brain stem **94–5**, **96–8**, 143
suckling, prolactin levels and 56, 139
supranuclear mechanisms, eye movements 47, 139
sweating, insulinoma 60
sympathetic nerve supply
    bladder control 88–9, 142–3
    pons 96, 143
    recurrent paraganglioma and 23
Synacthen test 50, 58
syphilis 16, 97
syringomyelia **87–8**, 142–3

tachycardia
    paroxysmal ventricular 131
    sinus, causes 10, 11, 136
Takayasu's disease 16–17
tall stature 66, 140
telangiectases 76, 77, 141
    hereditary haemorrhagic **76–7**, 141
temporal arteritis 16
temporomandibular joint disorder 103
tendons 13
testes
    atrophy 99, 144
    biopsy 63
    Klinefelter's syndrome 64, 140
testicular cancer 64, 140
testosterone 36, 138
    low level in primary hypopituitarism 58
    macroprolactinoma 55
tetralogy of Fallot 133, 146–7
thirst, Langerhans cell histiocytosis 28
Thomsen's disease 100
thoracic nerve root damage 97
thrombocytopenia, causes 125
thrombocytosis 120
thrombosis, polycythaemia rubra vera association 120–1
thrombotic thrombocytopenic purpura 77

thyroglobulin 44
thyroglossal cysts 44
thyroid gland, embryology 44, 138
thyroid hormones
  in hypopituitarism 58, 140
  metabolic effects 44–5
  synthesis 44
thyroid microsomal autoantibodies 46
thyroid-stimulating hormone (TSH) 140
  hypothyroidism 43
  low level in autoimmune thyrotoxicosis 46
  raised levels 40, 43
thyrotoxicosis, autoimmune **46–8**, 139
thyroxine 36, 46, 138
tidal volume 116, 145
tiredness
  Addison's disease 49
  polycythaemia rubra vera 120
  primary biliary cirrhosis 79
  primary hypopituitarism 58–9, 140
  see also lethargy
T lymphocytes 140
  CD4, HIV receptor 2, 135
  sarcoid granulomas 115, 145
tongue, spasticity 85
total lung capacity 116, 145
toxoplasma encephalitis 135
Toxoplasma gondii 3, 135
transposition of the great vessels 133
trigeminal ganglion 91
trigeminal nerve
  anatomy 91
  palsy **90–1**, 143
trigeminal neuralgia 90–1
trigeminal sensory neuropathy 91
triglycerides, synthesis 53
trimethoprim–sulfamethoxazole 3
trinucleotide repeat expansion 100, 143
Trousseau's sign 41
truncoconal septum 133, 147
truncus arteriosus, persistent 133, 147
tryptophan 75
tuberculosis
  bone and joint involvement 7–8
  spinal **7–8**, 135
tumour markers 20
Turner's syndrome 10, 130

ulcerative colitis 118
ulnar nerve, damage 93
upper motor neurone
  degenerative loss 86, 142
  paralysis in pseudobulbar palsy 135
urea 36
urinary continence, in motor neurone disease 142
urine
  alkaline 38
  calcium increase 38
  dark colour 31, 78
  inappropriately dilute 29

uveitis, anterior, in sarcoidosis 111

vagus nerve, dorsal motor nucleus 11, 136
Valsalva's manoeuvre 89, 142
vasculitis 16
  granulomatous 16
  Henoch–Schönlein purpura 77
  necrotizing 15, 16
  types 16–17
vasomotor centre 11, 135
vasopressin 29–30, 36
  secretion and role 29–30
  synthesis 29, 137
velocardiofacial syndrome 10
ventricular septal defects 131, 133, 147
vertebral collapse, spinal tuberculosis 8, 135
vertebral disorders, spinal tuberculosis 8
vertebrobasilar arterial supply 143
vessel wall disorders 76, 77, 125, 141, 146
vestibular nerve damage, nystagmus due to 95
vestibular nuclei, nystagmus due to 95
vestibulocochlear nerve (VIIIth cranial nerve), nystagmus due to 95
vibration 135
vision, blurred 55
vision impairment
  cerebral sarcoidosis 111–13, 145
  macroprolactinoma 55–7, 71, 139
visual aura 60
visual field loss, pituitary tumours 57, 139
visual pathway, lesions 47
vital capacity 116, 145
vitamin B_{12}, decreased levels in AIDS 2
vitamins, fat-soluble 53
vitamin supplements, in carcinoid tumours 74
vitiligo 40
voice, nasal, in dermatomyositis 4–6, 135
vomiting
  blood *see* haematemesis
  'coffee grounds' 123
  intracranial tumours 83
  recurrent paraganglioma 23–4, 137
  renal tubular acidosis 37
von Hippel–Lindau syndrome 88
von Reckinghausen's syndrome (neurofibromatosis) **21–2**, 136–7
von Willebrand's disease **123–5**, 146
von Willebrand's factor 123, 146

water deprivation test 137
weakness *see* muscle weakness
Wegener's granulomatosis **15–17**, 136
weight gain, insulinoma 60, 140
weight loss
  Addison's disease 49
  motor neurone disease 85
  primary biliary cirrhosis 78–80
Wilson's disease **81–2**, 142
Wolff–Parkinson–White syndrome **126–8**, 146

XXY genotype 63, 140

Instructions for use of CD

1. Install the CD according to the instructions given in the booklet.
2. First screen: select whether you want to view the cases randomly (click central icon) or by system (click desired system icon).
3. Play the video clip(s).
4. Think about the differential diagnosis.
5. Look at the case notes in the book and read the basic science associated with the case.
6. Try the multiple choice questions either on the CD or in the book.
7. The bottom left icon reveals useful diagrams for you to look at. (These are often extra diagrams that do not appear in the book.)

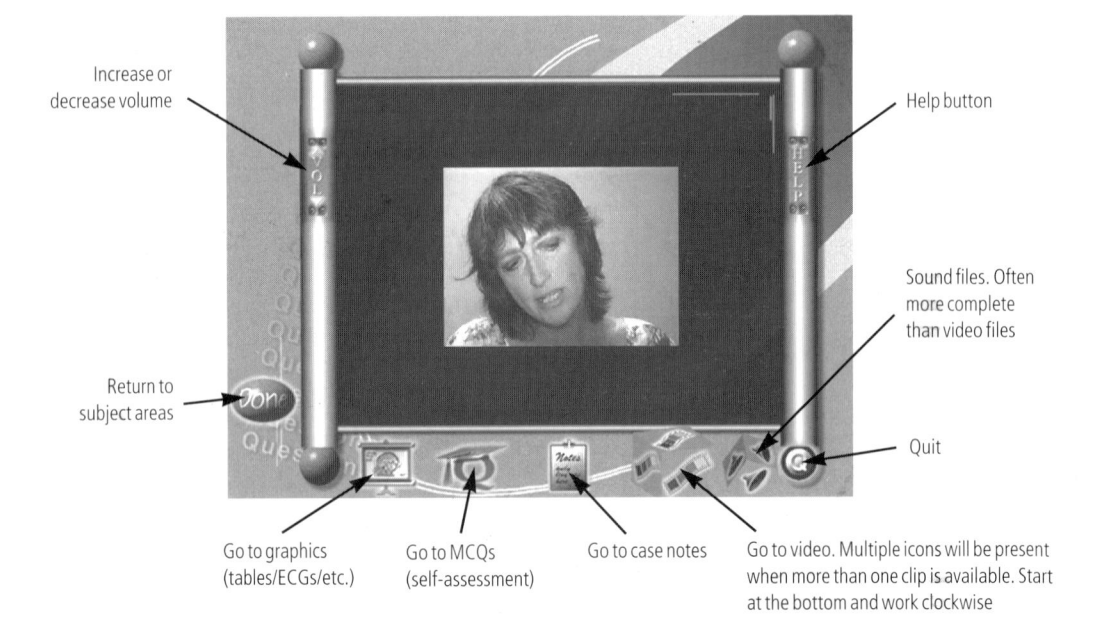

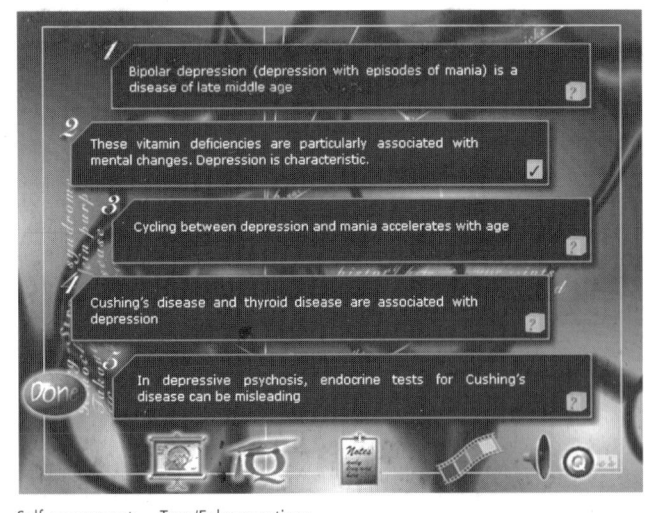

Note that the case resolution and basic science are NOT included on the CD, they are only in the book.

- Increase or decrease volume
- Help button
- Sound files. Often more complete than video files
- Return to subject areas
- Quit
- Go to graphics (tables/ECGs/etc.)
- Go to MCQs (self-assessment)
- Go to case notes
- Go to video. Multiple icons will be present when more than one clip is available. Start at the bottom and work clockwise

1. Bipolar depression (depression with episodes of mania) is a disease of late middle age
2. These vitamin deficiencies are particularly associated with mental changes. Depression is characteristic.
3. Cycling between depression and mania accelerates with age
4. Cushing's disease and thyroid disease are associated with depression
5. In depressive psychosis, endocrine tests for Cushing's disease can be misleading

Self-assessment — True/False questions